"There are no incurable diseases."
– Ann Wigmore

For every cooked food there is a raw version.

Dead cooked foods offer only death – not life.
Only living foods have the life-giving power
to heal from diseases and life-threatening
illnesses.

When one goes from cooked foods to
raw living foods, the Laws of Nature change.

The rules that apply to cooked foods
no longer work in the realm of living foods.
It is in this higher dimension of living
where healing begins.

The
Healing Power
Of
Living Foods

Linda Lamar Ruff, R.D.

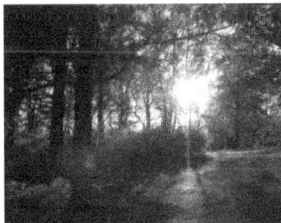

Vita Aeterna
Advanced Wellness Books

The information in this book is not intended to diagnose or prescribe. This information is only to enhance modern medicine - not replace it. Always consult with a physician or other qualified health care practitioner to diagnose, prescribe, or treat any illness or disease.

The author and publisher do not accept responsibility for any risk involved in the material or contents of this book. This responsibility belongs solely to the reader for no one but the reader knows how he or she best feels in his or her body. Therefore, it is the right of the reader to choose a lifestyle and treatment that is best for him or her. And always get a second opinion from a qualified health care professional before embarking upon any lifestyle change.

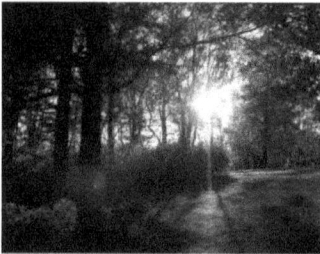

Vita Aeterna
Advanced Wellness Books

Published in the United States by Vita Aeterna Advanced Wellness Books, an imprint of Bird Brain Publishing, a division of Bird Brain Productions, LLC, Evansville, Indiana. www.birdbrainpublishing.com
PRINTED IN THE UNITED STATES OF AMERICA

Cover design and graphic art by Whitney Arvin

First Edition

ISBN-10: 1937668991
ISBN-13: 978-1-937668-99-0

To my father Byron Lamar

for leading me to this path

and

David McNeely

for making this journey possible.

Linda Lamar Ruff, R.D.

The
Healing Power
Of
Living Foods

By
Linda Lamar Ruff, R.D.

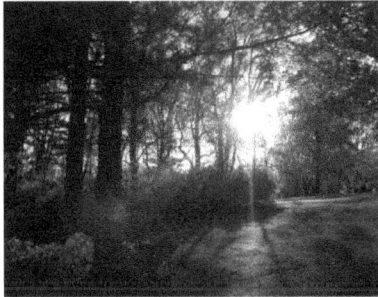

Vita Aeterna
Advanced Wellness Books
Evansville, Indiana

Table of Contents

Acknowledgements

I am grateful to the people who chose to help others by allowing me to use their case histories.

I wish to thank those who gave me permission to use their recipes.

I am thankful to my publisher John for believing in my book and my sister Bonnie, Mark, and Christopher for their editing support. I wish to thank those who encouraged me to write the book and supported me through the process.

I thank Susan, Leola, and Lalita for their valuable support and feedback. Most importantly, I am grateful that they chose to carry on Dr. Ann's work so that I and others can grow in healthy, quality lives while Mother Earth heals.

I appreciate my family for patiently waiting for me to complete the book.

Most of all, I pray rich blessings upon those who are passionately working to restore peace and healing to Mother Earth and all life within Her bosom.

Foreword

My name is Leola A. Brooks and I am the co-director of the Ann Wigmore Natural Health Institute in Puerto Rico. I have been connected to raw and living foods for over thirty years.

Dr. Ann Wigmore was the founder of the Institute and of the Living Foods Lifestyle® and before she died, she selected both Lalita Salas and myself to continue her legacy. Part of my continuing her mission is to encourage others to share the health benefits of eating raw and living foods and I support the benefits that Linda's book may bring to others.

Linda Ruff was introduced to wheatgrass and a new way of eating at the Ann Wigmore Natural Health Institute in 1995 but seemed to know intuitively that the Living Foods Lifestyle® was the doorway to good health. While at the Institute, Linda was taught that this lifestyle requires taking responsibility for your own health and wellbeing. She learned that Dr. Ann Wigmore worked with almost every disease imaginable and that she found two distinct causes.

1. Toxicity
2. Deficiency

She learned that we must remove the toxins and supply the body with the missing elements in order to eliminate the deficiency and the disease. We must bring balance to the body with proper nutrition.

As a registered dietitian, Linda's training at the Institute as a student, and later as an instructor, allowed her to see firsthand the challenges that people face when eating habits are changed from cooked foods to raw and living foods. She interviewed a large number of students about their health issues and why they had chosen the Ann Wigmore Natural Health Institute on their pathway to recovery.

Whenever prospective students and guests call me to ask if anyone with their particular illness has ever attended the Institute, I recall the many people that have visited over the years and my response is yes.

I was delighted to read case histories and stories in Linda's book, *The Healing Power of Living Foods*. You will be delighted as well. Linda has also taken the basics of the Living Foods Lifestyle®, adapted it to her culinary taste, and presented information in a new and personal way.

Lalita and I are grateful that Linda's book acknowledges Dr. Ann Wigmore for her work in founding the Living Foods Lifestyle® and wish her well with her book.

Leola Brooks
Co-Director of the Ann Wigmore Natural Health Institute

Introduction

Not long ago a journalist attended a lecture of mine on raw foods and wrote about it in the newspaper. While family, friends, and neighbors were impressed with the article, I was very disappointed - the healing powers of raw and living foods were not mentioned.

Then a message came to me: "No one will ever write about raw and living foods like you will. They can't."

I realized the veracity of this message. Unless people have experienced a totally raw living foods diet along with a detoxification program, they cannot write about the energy, life, and restorative healing powers within.

After all, they do not have the disappearance of aches, pains, wrinkles, warts, and moles from eating cooked foods. They have not seen the appearance of a smooth, flawless complexion full of the beautiful, pure glow of life coming through. They have not been so rested and energized that, the second they open their eyes in the morning, they enthusiastically leap out of bed to charge into daily tasks. They have not noticed their days growing longer and getting much work done with time to spare at the end of the day. Eating cooked foods does not provide the life and vitality surging through their veins with each waking moment. They do not feel vibrancy and strength coursing through their bodies with each step.

When experiencing the Living Foods Lifestyle®, the eyes become bright and sparkly, and the vision clears. As one sees better, the head feels lighter, and mental clarity sharpens. On a deeper level, intuition becomes honed, and vision, wisdom, and assurance for life's path become clear from a cleansed body. One experiences the joy and peace in one's soul when the body is cleansed and made whole. No words will ever convey the profound magic of life flowing from within the body to all and everything that comes into contact with it unless one has experienced this powerful lifestyle.

Unfortunately, today we are robbed of this legacy of health and vitality designed for us by the Divine Creator. Instead of feeling refreshed and energized after eating a meal, all too many times we feel sluggish and drowsy and need a nap afterward. This is because "the wonders of chemistry" have used heat, additives, and chemicals and altered the molecular structure of foods faster than the body can genetically adapt.

Therefore, the body does not recognize it as food. Instead the imitation or "pseudo-foods" become toxins that the body must throw off. Energies then must be taken from other parts of the body, causing fatigue and drowsiness, to do something with the ingested matter. With time the body finds it harder to eliminate this material. When the digestive tract becomes too tired and weak to eliminate it, it becomes easier to store the matter in weak areas of the body to become moles, tumors, excess body weight, and health issues. Hence, sickness and disease build up in the body creating malfunctions throughout.

Those who cling to cooked foods go through life tired and drained from the aches, pains, and sickness that lifeless pseudo-foods bring until getting through the day becomes a chore. Then they struggle just to make it through the hour, let alone accomplish what needs to be done throughout the day. In short, our devitalized, nutritionally-devoid food supply is draining us and dragging us down into a lower dimension of living until we are literally dying before the last breath departs from the body.

But why do people persist in eating cooked foods? While it is easy to eat raw foods, it is hard *not* to eat cooked foods. It means we would have to give up our favorite foods that we *think* "keep us going." Hence, our soft drinks, pastries, meat, or whatever it is that holds us back actually becomes an addiction and keeps us from moving forward into a joyful, vibrant life. While many on a cooked food diet eat some raw foods just because raw food tastes so flavorful and sumptuous, they will never know true healing and life by doing partly raw each day – let alone write about it.

In the early 1990's few books were written on raw foods. Since then, many books with raw recipes are available until the recipes appear to be similar. But I know of none that tells or explains the magical healing powers of raw and living foods seen in practice.

Therefore, I wrote this book with case histories of healing observed first hand both in my practice and at the Ann Wigmore Natural Health Institute in Puerto Rico. Also I have included some history on how Dr. Ann Wigmore helped promote the raw foods movement by virtue of her work. I declare each and every story in this book to be true. Only the details of the individuals in the case histories have been altered to protect their confidentiality.

Also included are menus and recipes that restore and promote good health. When followed consistently, the body turns around to life and healing. Perhaps my writings will create a greater understanding of the power inherent in raw veganism and the Living Foods Lifestyle[®] so that healing and peace will prevail on Mother Earth.

Chapter 1
Mother Nature Knows Best

She was only a teen-ager when driving the wagon to deliver bread in Middleboro, Massachusetts. The horse had endured abuse during its life and was easily frightened.

One day a noisy "horseless carriage" pulled out in front of the horse. This so frightened the horse that it bolted, and when it had stopped, the wagon lay on her legs, pinning her to the ground. As the confused horse tried to move out of its predicament, the wagon gradually crept up her body and cut the air off to her lungs.

Although a distant dog down the road could not see the accident, it instinctively knew she was in trouble. It barked and barked an alarm until its owner followed it to the scene of the accident. There the man literally lifted the heavy wooden wagon off of her body by himself.

Later at the hospital Ann Wigmore learned that both of her legs were broken down near the ankles, but instead of healing, the skin on her legs turned an ominous color, and gangrene set in.

The doctors insisted that her legs be amputated below the knees to save her life, but she obstinately refused, much to the wrath of her father. After all, during World War I in their small Lithuanian village, she had seen her grandmother use diet and packs of herbs and grasses to nurse many soldiers with gangrene back to health, and she felt the amputations were unnecessary.

Fortunately for her, she was now "of age" at eighteen years old; her father could not force her to undergo the surgery. So she was released from the hospital as a "hopeless case" and sent home to die.

While her family waited for her to die from certain death that slowly crept up her legs, her uncle carried her to a bench in the grass of the yard each morning before he left for work. There she basked in the sunlight and nibbled on flowers and grasses throughout the day.

Feeling excruciating pain from the gangrene and loneliness as family shunned her, she befriended a white puppy, who lay in the shade under her bench where she reclined.

One sunny morning he scrambled up on her bench, careful not to touch her painful legs. As he started to lick her legs, she impulsively reached to stop him lest he become sick, but suddenly her grandmother's words of wisdom jumped into her thoughts.

"Instinct-guided creatures, left to themselves, do not make mistakes." So she allowed "Little Angel" to lick the pus-filled flesh on her thin legs.

Amazingly, the pain in her legs started easing, and she managed to sit for the first time. From then on Little Angel came to lick her legs twice a day like clockwork.

While it took several months, the stench from the gangrene slowly faded, the green flesh turned to pink again, her broken bones healed very well, and she walked again much to the anger of her father. Thus, two dogs helped save her life, and many years later she ran in marathons (1, 2).

Like Ann, my grandfather had a similar story. As a boy, he cut his leg open with a corn knife during harvest, and gangrene set in. After a few visits, the family doctor shook his head and said there was nothing more he could do. He did, however, ask if there was a dog around. When told yes, the doctor said to let the dog lick his wound.

With time, the gangrene went away. Grampa grew up to have a large family, and two generations later here am I.

While these two stories may seem phenomenal, they just go to show that healing can come from many unexpected sources. Also Mother Nature provides healing for every kind of ailment on this planet, and just as our forefathers relied upon Her, perhaps we should tap more often into Her boundless resources.

Chapter 2
Raw Foods Case Histories

Nodules of the Lungs

He was a 50-year-old nurse with two children from St. Croix. After many tests, the doctor felt there might be nodules in his lungs but wanted to run another test "just to be sure."

By this time the nurse was tired of tests and decided to come to the Institute instead. His uncle had done the program before and accompanied him to help.

When he arrived, he was very weak and found it difficult to climb the stairs. The first week he had an unproductive cough. By the end of the first week, his cough was productive.

Ten days later while walking to my apartment overlooking the ocean, I heard someone calling, "Linda! Linda!"

When I looked up, he was lying in the sunlight on a picnic table next to the student building. He yelled, "Linda! Come here quick!"

When I walked over, he was very excited.

"My pain. It's gone! It's gone! Well, maybe just a dull thud. But! the pain is gone!" He was jubilant.

I applauded him and explained that for many students on the program the pain from tumors and other cancers will leave in just a matter of days.

By his last class, he was feeling much stronger. He left the Institute imbued with life.

Rectal Tumor

The 41-year-old doctor had difficulty sitting through his first class. He crossed and uncrossed his legs every minute or two. The next day he called me aside to tell me that he had a tumor next to his rectum and might not be able to sit through a whole class.

About one and a half weeks after his arrival, a director of the Institute, who was sitting with the doctor on the veranda, called to me. When I went over, the doctor was crying, and the director asked me to speak with him.

I listened to him as he poured his heart out in tears over personal matters. "And here I've got this painful tumor." He was terribly frightened.

With his permission I laid my hand on his arm. I then said, "While I do not know about your case, many people with tumors find their pain starting to disappear by the second week."

Immediately he sat up. His eyes opened wide, and his tears dried up. He said, "I used to cross my legs every three or four minutes, but now I only cross them in about twenty!"

Suddenly he jumped up and went on his way. He knew he was going to be okay after all.

Thyroid Cancer

She was 39 years old and from Haiti. When she came down with thyroid cancer, she was a stockbroker in New York City. She then gave up the high-stress world and went to the Institute, where she was an accomplished yoga instructor.

When I first met her, she had what appeared to be an "Adam's apple," or bump on her throat. She was constantly eating the green energy soup or wallowing the wheatgrass juice in her mouth. She spoke little, if any, and only nodded her head.

Two years later I saw her, among many yoga poses, standing on her hands with her legs wrapped around her body and looking very much like a large duck. Her "Adam's apple" was gone, and she spoke and laughed freely as she went about her day. One would never know she once had a life-threatening illness.

Type 1 Diabetes

She was a type 1 diabetic with a dress shop in Illinois. At thirty years of age she had divorced and become blind at the same time. At thirty-eight years of age, she attended the Institute with her seeing-eye dog to learn of the Living Foods Lifestyle®.

The first week during the program, she found herself urinating frequently, so she checked to see if she was going into ketosis. Her test came out negative, indicating her body was releasing trapped fluid. But her blood sugar levels became erratic. By the end of that week, she and the naturopath at the Institute determined that the fermented liquid called rejuvelac, which provides probiotics and other beneficial properties, was creating sugar imbalances. She then stopped drinking it but had no problems when eating foods prepared with it.

By the end of the second week, not only were her blood sugar levels stable, but she had also reduced her insulin dosage by one-third to one-half the amount. Years later, although not totally raw, she was amazed to find that she did not have neuropathy, nephropathy, and other debilitating diseases that often accompany diabetics on the standard American diet.

Type 2 Diabetes

He was a retired businessman from Puerto Rico, who practiced yoga religiously. He also had type 2 diabetes.

At sixty-two years of age he came to the Institute to do the program. After fifteen days, he reached into the refrigerator for his last vial of insulin only to drop and shatter it on the tile floor. At first, he felt horrified that his last dosage was gone, but then his yoga philosophy kicked in, and he stopped and thought: perhaps this was a message to him that he no longer needed his insulin.

Instead of running for a prescription refill, he went without only to discover his blood sugar levels were within normal range. He told me, "In fact, when I take my insulin, it makes my sugar levels go up." So after that, he practiced the lifestyle and went without insulin.

CAUTION: Many have stabilized their blood sugar levels without insulin simply by adopting the Living Foods Lifestyle®. But *never* attempt such an undertaking without the guidance of a health care practitioner experienced in diabetes and the Living Foods Lifestyle®. Serious results could occur, including coma and death, without a qualified professional to monitor and assist in such an endeavor.

Obesity

He was a forty-one-year-old nurse over six feet tall, who weighed six hundred pounds and was on medication for cholesterol and diabetes. Two years prior to his counseling session, he had fallen on the job with a heart attack.

Fortunately for him, it was April, and summer was on its way with an abundance of fresh produce. I told him to drink lots of pure clean water and to eat many fresh fruits, vegetables, and melons.

By August of that year, he had lost one hundred pounds.

By October, with his doctor's supervision, he was off his cholesterol medication.

In November he was down to 450 pounds, and his blood pressure was down from 140/106 to 130/60.

By December of that same year, his doctor took him off his diabetes medication and said, "There's no reason to keep you on it."

She was thirty-eight years old and an office worker in Puerto Rico. One of her co-workers had lost weight while at the Institute, so she came to see if the program would work for her.

When I first saw her, her large midriff stuck out further than her ample chest.

Two weeks later, her midriff had receded considerably, and her chest was standing out further than her midriff.

Needless to say, she was pleased with the results when she left.

Cardiovascular Disease

He was from Indiana with a career in professional negotiations and labor relations. While he had become vegetarian, he compensated for his lack of meat by increasing his consumption of dairy foods, which were heavy with cholesterol and saturated fats. By fifty-nine, his countless days of travel in the Midwestern states, eating out, and stress had rewarded him with triple by-pass surgery.

After his surgery, he did not find it to be very much fun, so he asked his cardiologist, "How long before I go through this again?"

The cardiologist replied, "Five years, if you don't change your ways."

He then decided he did not want to endure another such surgery. Two years later, he traveled to the Institute. A year after adopting the lifestyle, his cardiologist stated that his numbers were completely normal and released him.

Irritable Bowel Symptoms

She was a health care para-professional who at 63 years of age suffered severe abdominal pain and swelling on her right side along with symptoms of bloating, gas, loose stools, and other colon disturbances similar to irritable bowel syndrome, colitis, and Crohn's disease. For years she had suffered the pain intermittently which was gradually worsening. She chose to try living foods and supplements to improve her condition. She particularly liked how the raw onion kraut (see recipe in chapter 13) soothed her digestive tract.

In the meantime she knew someone with identical symptoms on the same side of the body at the same time who opted for medical treatment. At the emergency room the acquaintance was immediately wheeled away to surgery for a colostomy to prevent rupturing and death. The surgery left the acquaintance ill and weak and was later followed by a second surgery.

On the other hand, after four months of doing living foods, the 63-year-old lady's pain, weakness, and swelling disappeared. She was grateful she had chosen living foods to improve her health.

Chronic Infection

He was thirty-seven-years-old from the Caribbean island of Tortola. For two years he had suffered with an ear infection, and for two years he had fought it with antibiotics. Yet no matter what he tried, nothing worked. He had heard of the Ann Wigmore Natural Health Institute, so out of desperation he decided to go there and give the program a try.

For the first few days, the pain intensified. An earache kept him awake until two in the morning, so he used pain medicine to sleep. By the fifth day, however, he thought his earache might be diminishing. By the seventh day the ear infection that he had suffered with for two years was totally gone. He was elated!

While he was there, he decided to stop smoking as a surprise for his family upon his return home.

Arthritis

She was a real estate agent from California in her early fifties. Crippled with arthritis, she walked with a beautifully carved wooden cane topped with a shiny brass handle. She stated she awakened in the mornings very stiff and had to work her body just to move out of bed.

Five or six years prior to her arrival at the Institute, she had gone on crutches to another raw foods institute in California and rid herself of arthritis in a couple of weeks. However, she had not followed their program after her departure. Instead, she ate what whim and convenience dictated, and with time the arthritis returned.

After two weeks in Puerto Rico, she became impatient because she was not healing fast enough on the program to suit herself. She felt the juicing program used at the institute in California worked much faster. But she opted to stay another week in Puerto Rico anyway.

As the third week moved forward, she was getting very concerned. Her arthritis still had not left.

However, right before her departure she was laughing and hugging everyone in the office. She stated, "I walked into the Institute with a cane, and now I am walking out without one! I'll be back!"

Asthma

She was eleven years old in Wisconsin when she awakened in the middle of the night gasping to get air into her painful lungs. Later that night at the hospital her diagnosis was asthma. The very next day her brothers and sisters got very angry with her and would not speak to her for some time because they had to get rid of their pets. Testing showed that she was allergic to cats, dogs, feathers, dust, and certain grasses.

The asthma haunted her throughout her life. During her childhood she was rushed to the emergency room many times. She had to stay outside in the yard at the birthday parties of friends with house pets. If she tried to spend the night, she always came home sick. She could not vacuum or dust. As an adult, horseback riding sent her to the hospital with the cornea swelling over the iris and pupil of her eyes until she could not see. While she used her illness as an excuse to skip class or get out of trouble, she still felt the asthma was not worth it.

She could go nowhere without her steroid pills. While they helped her to breathe, her body could not tolerate them, and they made her seriously ill. Yet she had no choice but to use them. Then at about age twenty she discovered that she did not need her pills if she drank a certain herbal tea when she sensed an impending attack. With the help of the tea, she got off all medication and started drifting toward natural healing. But she still avoided any asthma triggers.

At 39 years of age she discovered and embraced raw foods religiously. More than ten years later, she was astounded to find that she could live in the same house with two cats without suffering any ill effects with breathing.

Multiple Schlerosis

One day while back in the harvest room getting sprouts ready for that day's meals, I heard much shouting and laughter up front in the student building. It seemed a beloved celebrity had returned after a long absence, and much celebration was in the air.

Later at dinner I conversed with a lady sitting next to me. She looked at another lady across the table from us and stopped dead in the middle of her sentence.

"Is that you?" she asked incredulously.

"Yes," replied the lady sitting next to her mother across from us.

The lady next to me stared at her and said, "I didn't know you!"

The daughter again replied, "I know you didn't. I was gaunt," and she sucked in her cheeks to demonstrate how emaciated she had been.

She then showed us a three-year-old picture of herself as a gray-headed, emaciated woman who had, with her mother's help, come to the Institute.

At the time of the picture, she was a thirty-two-year-old lady, who had worked for the owner of a yacht until she was diagnosed with multiple schlerosis. Wine and cheese, which she loved, had been the mainstay of her diet. But that changed when she came to the Institute and learned to follow the program.

Now she was a vibrant thirty-five-year-old lady with a short, beautifully coiffed hairdo that was once more her natural auburn color. She no longer needed assistance from her mother to get around throughout the day, and one would never dream she had once been a debilitated old woman.

As we ate, the lady next to me asked, "What do you think restored your health?"

The daughter across the table stated, "The diet here."

The lady next to me plied, "Are you sure?"

The lady across the dining room table responded, "Yes." But she paused and reflected.

"Well, the yoga also helped," she added. "Either I was too weak or it was too painful to get into the positions like everyone else. But my instructor stayed with me and helped me get into the positions, and now she is a good friend of mine.

"But both the diet and yoga are what restored my health."

Lyme Disease

She was a thirty-six-year-old schoolteacher, who decided to take off for a full year. She bought a shell to go on the back of her pick-up truck and toured the United States. One morning after sleeping out all night, she awakened to find herself covered with ticks.

Later at the doctor's office, Lyme disease was confirmed. The doctor wanted to start with the least expensive regimen for several thousand dollars, and if that did not help, he would move to the next level of treatment which was more expensive.

Perhaps the young lady no longer had health insurance, but for whatever reason she decided to try a different approach. She traveled to the Institute where she learned how to strengthen her immune system.

While it took six months of practicing the new lifestyle, her health became completely restored, and the Lyme disease totally disappeared.

Parkinson's Disease

The first few times I attended the Institute, I was literally awestruck by the healings I saw. I would feel that nothing else would amaze me, but then another astonishing healing would manifest itself, and once again I would be amazed. Apparently I was not the only one who felt astonished by these miracles as the following case history shows.

The red-headed young man from Ireland who worked in the kitchen ran out of the building onto the veranda. "Did you see him?" he asked incredulously. "Did you see him when he left?"

Others seemed to pay no heed. After all, healings were commonplace at the Institute.

I responded, "Why?"

The Irishman replied, awestruck. He simply could not believe the difference in the elderly man from the time he had arrived until he left.

The elderly man was a retired 73-year-old from Israel who once owned many cab companies in New York City. He also had Parkinson's Disease.

When he arrived, he trembled and had a shuffled gait. When he left, he walked out of the student building without assistance. One would never know he had any disease at all.

Dyslexia

She was a thirty-nine-year-old freelance photographer from California who had been one hundred percent raw for two years.

Upon her arrival while enroute from the airport to the Institute, I asked about her experiences with the raw lifestyle. She stated her dyslexia had totally corrected itself and disappeared.

"Do you ever get sick?" I asked.

"No," she replied. Then she caught herself.

"While I've never been sick, I did get a red rash about six months after eating totally raw. It started on my stomach and worked its way up my chest to my neck and then on up and out of my head. It never itched or hurt nor was it uncomfortable in any way. But I've never experienced any sickness or health issues."

Motor Skill Degeneration

The first time I saw her, her husband was patiently holding her walker on the stair landing while she tried pulling herself up by the rail, her exercise for the day.

She was a forty-two-year-old accountant with a successful CPA business. Unfortunately, she had to dispose of her business because her motor skills were deteriorating to the point that she could not talk plain or function. Her husband, a manager in a company, suffered with migraine headaches.

She and a friend had played cards every Wednesday night "without fail for twenty-two years," but she gave that up as her ability to function had waned. Fortunately, the friend had been to the Ann Wigmore Natural Health Institute and was "wowed" by what she discovered there. The friend told the accountant and her husband about the Institute and tried to convince them to try the program.

Neither was interested; besides the accountant was fearful of flying. Yet the friend persisted without let-up until, at great length, the accountant and her husband relented.

The accountant had to be boarded onto the plane on a stretcher. She panicked every time the plane hit an air pocket. Her card-playing friend, who was sitting next to her, just laughed, patted her hand, and told her to relax.

Four days after their arrival at the Institute, I was walking on the veranda, where the accountant and her friend were once again playing cards. As I walked past, I suddenly stopped dead in my tracks. Wait a minute, I thought to myself. They are playing cards!

I backed up in my tracks just enough to see the friend duck behind her cards and grin widely at me. She held up four fingers and quietly mouthed the words to me, "Only four days! Only four days!" Then it was her turn to play.

I continued to watch as they played. While the accountant still could not talk, she was confidently slapping down those cards and making snappy vocal noises that she herself understood. Again the friend ducked behind the cards and mouthed the words to me, "She won't admit it's the diet."

By the second week, the accountant was swiftly shoving her walker everywhere she went. Many noticed and remarked upon it. By the end of the two-weeks program, she had improved dramatically.

A couple of years later I saw the friend, who returned many times with her family. I asked her how the accountant was doing.

"She's in a nursing home.

Stunned, I asked, "What?"

The friend slowly repeated, "She's in a nursing home."

"What happened?" I asked.

The friend stated, "Her husband and I asked her, 'Well, what do you think?' We were shocked when she replied that the food did not work."

The friend slowly continued, "Linda, after boarding the plane for Puerto Rico on a stretcher, she *walked* off that plane back home *without* her walker, but she refused to admit that the foods helped her."

I reflected for a moment and then asked, "What about her husband?"

"Oh," she replied, "he continued with the program and got rid of his migraines. But she refused the program, so she's in a nursing home." She shrugged.

Sometimes we simply have to love people enough to allow them their choices and trust that all between them and the Divine Creator is as it should be.

Feet Discoloration

Although his field was in nursing, he had recently retired as a school administrator in Philadelphia. Just when he had planned to relax and enjoy himself, he was diagnosed with cancer. While he had gone to a medical doctor, he wanted to try a different approach first.

When he arrived at the Institute, his gold-rimmed eyeglasses against his dark skin looked very healthy, so I told him he had fine skin.

He said, "No!"

I asked, "Why not?"

He pointed to his feet. Above the ankles the skin was red. Below the ankles his feet were blue, and his toes were purple.

Near the end of the two-weeks program, I asked how he felt about the lifestyle.

"I am skeptical. But! I am going to stay another two weeks."

At the end of the next week while whale-watching on a boat, I asked him how he felt.

"I'm still skeptical. *But* my doctor and I are going to have a talk."

By the end of his last week, I asked what he thought of the program.

"It works!"

"Why do you say so?" I asked.

"Look!" Then he pointed to his feet.

The skin above the ankles was its natural color, and red had replaced the blue and purple colors on his feet. He was jubilant.

He emphatically stated, "My doctor and I are going to have a talk, and we are going to come to an understanding."

He left with hope and enthusiasm. Although I never heard any more about his cancer, he came back to the Institute with his family several times. He enjoyed his retirement after all.

Hearing Loss

He was a retired eighty-year-old building contractor from Connecticut. His hearing had faded and was so far gone that he communicated mostly with his wife and did little participation himself in classes.

One morning into the second week of the program, he awakened to the sound of a low roar. He thought to himself, "What is that?"

Then it occurred to him that he was hearing the roar of the ocean.

Mercury Toxicity

While her field was history, she was on leave of absence from public relations work in a winery in central California. As she spoke, she put her fingers in her ears to endure head pain caused by bursts of thunder from the afternoon tropical storm.

She had no medical history. She grew up on fish one to two times a week and drank two to three glasses of milk a day. Since she was a thin child, her mother always provided her with an egg and milk mixture to "fill me out." She had only two cavities in her whole life, but her cholesterol was high at eleven years of age.

Eight years prior to her arrival at the Institute, she had switched from dairy to soy and rice milks. Three years later she had colon hydrotherapy every one or two months. She ran, swam, and played tennis. What with good diet, exercise, and colon cleansing, she felt she should be extremely healthy. Yet health issues kept her from leading a productive life.

Three years prior to her arrival at the Institute the loud blast of speakers created endless tinnitus (ringing in the ears). She suffered from hyperacusis (extreme sensitivity to sound), which caused pain and swelling in her inner ear.

Photophobia was disrupting her life. She could no longer fly an airplane because looking directly into the sun created floaters and black spots that hampered her vision. Flashing lights created terrible frontal lobe headaches and prevented her from driving at night, watching television, or using a computer. She suffered recurring headaches, particularly from sudden movement, such as trying to catch something as it fell.

She had joint pains of the knees, feet, elbows, shoulders, and particularly in the wrists and hands, making it too painful to play the guitar. She experienced burning sensations in her hands and feet and did not dare walk barefoot in the shower because of cleaning solutions. Her eyelashes quivered uncontrollably, and an abrupt head movement brought about "an occasional heart tremor." Her skin was ruddy red, and her eyes were bloodshot.

Needless to say, she felt fatigued and depressed. She felt others saw her as reclusive or strange because she spent most of her time in her room. Yet she could not endure the pain caused by the high-pitched voices and laughter of the women. At 27 years of age, she stated, "I am simply too young to be this sick."

Her first step was to choose "an open-minded M.D." Tests showed that she was very low in toxic metals except for mercury which was high. Her doctor wanted her to have a stool analysis, but she was tired of the many tests and refused.

She was put on chelating agents and had her mercury fillings removed. She also used a drawing clay in which she soaked her hands. When she lifted her hands out, she could see tiny black beads the size of pores on her skin. But it was a slow process, and the detoxification program only heightened her symptoms.

Next she tried a health retreat in California with a program similar to the Institute's and had a positive experience. Then she left the bustle of the freeway there for the peace and healing of the ocean at the Institute in Puerto Rico.

Beginning the second day after arrival, she experienced uncontrollable tremors in her hands, fingers, and wrists. She suffered extreme sensitivity to car exhaust and dust from the air and ocean. Her feet burned, and her lungs felt pained and heavy. She had to work harder just to get air into her lungs.

She could not watch the videos during class instruction because of the headaches from the flashing screen. She could not hold a cell phone without pain coursing from her hand up to her shoulder and head.

After two weeks at the Institute, her thin frame had gone down ten to fifteen pounds but was now plateaued. She did not eat the papayas, dates, bananas, or other heavenly tropical fruits. *But* she did notice her headaches and photophobia were not as severe.

Nearly four weeks after her arrival, she still suffered from sensitivity to bright lights, tinnitus, car exhaust, and dust. As we spoke, she had to look down at the ground instead of into my eyes because the sun was toward her face.

She *did*, however, notice some improvements. The outbreak of pimples and rash on her chest were gone along with the heaviness in her lungs.

Her hyperacusis was both "up and down" in intensity. While she had experienced worsening joint pain in her legs, arms, and ankles the first three or four weeks at the Institute, she noticed the pain was drastically reduced and no longer woke her up of a night the last two weeks there. She became much surprised to find an old hip muscle injury improved while there.

Her face and skin became clear and white once more, and her eyes were no longer bloodshot. At this point, she had not tried playing the guitar to see how the joints in her hands and fingers would feel.

One week before leaving, she implemented one last thing into her detox program each day. She "snorted" two eyedroppers of wheatgrass juice into each nostril and cleansed her eyes with the juice. As she lowered her head between her knees, she could feel the juice going down into her sinuses, behind her eyes, and down into the frontal part of her head. She could feel "things loosening up." She felt pain in her sinuses and then snorted and coughed up blood, which was not from her lungs.

In a day or two, she developed a rash on the left side of her face. It was then that she noticed that throughout this healing crisis, her left eye and ear had been the most troublesome area with more pronounced symptoms.

After a few days of expectoration, her head felt "lighter, freer, clearer," and her headaches improved drastically. She felt that the mercury vapors that had gone to her sinuses when her fillings were removed were now clearing out.

At the end of her six-weeks stay, I found her to be very optimistic and hating to leave the Institute. She felt her body had adapted very well to the Living Foods program – "just like Mother's milk." She stated, "It's only six weeks, so it will take longer to get my body fully detoxed of mercury." She now ate some heavenly tropical fruits for breakfast and was no longer experiencing burning feet and lungs. She actually found herself "enjoying" running on the beach.

But the "biggies" were that her ears, eyes, and headaches had "improved a lot!" While the discomfort and pain of cleansing and healing had *not* been easy, she had disciplined herself to persevere through the program. Now she was feeling "pretty darn good." With the clearing of her head, her sense of well-being returned, and she gained insight into her life. She could now see what direction she wanted to take in her career. She now felt confident that she had her health built up enough to carry her through life's future challenges.

As I drove her to the airport for her departure, she stated that out of all the many things she did, she felt that "snorting" the wheatgrass juice brought the quickest and best results of all. She planned to purchase wheatgrass back in California until she could move to a place where she could grow it herself.

Chapter 3
What Are Raw and Living Foods?

The people in the above case histories restored their health from sickness and disease by following the Living Foods Lifestyle® which cleared dirt, debris, and toxins out of the body so that the vital life force in raw and living foods could enter in and begin the healing process. Dr. Ann Wigmore stated that the foods must be organic (grown in rich healthy soil devoid of chemicals and preservatives and not genetically modified).

Raw foods are whole foods that have not been heated above $110°$ Fahrenheit, pasteurized, or irradiated. Any temperature higher than that changes the molecular structure of food and kills off the vital life force within. These foods are in the form that they were grown, such as the apple that is eaten right after being picked off the tree.

Stop and think about a raw pea that has been picked fresh from the vine in the garden and shelled fresh from the pod. When it is planted and watered, a green sprout will grow up out of the soil in a matter of days and continue to grow into more vines and pods full of peas.

On the other hand, if instead of planting it, the pea is cooked at a temperature above $110°$ degrees and then planted in soil with water, that pea will not sprout and grow. Instead, it will rot and go back into the soil. Neither will it give life to the body after it has been cooked for food.

Living foods go one step further. Living foods are organic raw whole foods that are fermented to produce probiotics (the good bacteria), are teeming with food enzymes, and break protein down into amino acids, carbohydrates into simple sugars, and fats into fatty acids. Thus, living foods are predigested so that the body does not have to manufacture digestive enzymes to break down the complex molecules of chewed food when it reaches the gut. Instead, the gut can take a break and rest from its labors.

Living fermented foods are a very important part of the healing process. An example of a fermented food is raw cabbage that has been cultured into sauerkraut at room temperature. Other living foods are raw kim chee, raw cultured pickles and other vegetables, nut and seed cheeses and yogurts, and a fermented water called rejuvelac (see recipes in chapter 13).

Several studies show that a raw vegan diet is rich in probiotics and antioxidants and improves cases of rheumatoid arthritis and fibromyalgia (1,2,3,4). Raw and living foods are vital when the body is faced with a life-threatening illness. When fighting for its life, the body draws on all of its energies and vital life force to fight the invader, be it infection, cancer, or any other illness. Eating raw and living foods is like sending reinforcements to the site of the battle to fight the invading illness.

But when cooked foods enter the equation, the body has to withdraw its troops from the site of the infection, cancer, or illness to manufacture digestive enzymes and to help digest the cooked food in the gut. The withdrawn forces do not go back to the site of the illness until the food is digested. In the meantime, the illness can grow and damage the body while it is left unattended until the troops return to fight a now stronger invader.

Dead foods cannot bring life. Only raw living foods can provide the vital life force necessary to turn the body around from sickness and death to life and good health. This vital life force can be seen in Kirlian photography as an aura or energy field around a living thing, be it plant, animal, or human (5,6).

There are three types of enzymes that are linked to the vital life force: 1 - metabolic enzymes, which run the body's processes and functions; 2 - digestive enzymes consisting of proteases which digest protein, amylases which digest carbohydrates, and lipases which digest fats; and 3 - food enzymes found only in raw foods. Research shows that animals in the wild with a diet of totally raw foods have no concentrations of digestive enzymes in their saliva. On the other hand, digestive enzymes show up in the saliva of animals fed a diet of heated foods. The more cooked food in the diet, the greater the concentration of enzymes in the saliva (7).

Research also shows that the pancreas becomes enlarged on a cooked food diet because it has to manufacture digestive enzymes to compensate for missing food enzymes in cooked food (8). And just like tonsils enlarged from fighting an infection or a heart enlarged from cardiovascular disease, a pancreas becomes enlarged from the extra work of manufacturing digestive enzymes to digest cooked foods.

Many researchers, however, dispute this enzyme theory. Enzymes are made up of protein, which is broken down by hydrochloric acid and other digestive juices manufactured in the stomach. Therefore, many maintain that raw food enzymes are inactivated in the stomach and can have no value in the diet.

If indeed raw enzymes are rendered inactive from acids in the stomach, then something else in raw foods survives the stomach acids because the body experiences what no cooked food can bring - life! Only raw foods can restore the vital life force in a dying body.

Certainly Dr. Ann Wigmore, who established the Living Foods Lifestyle®, incorporated that life into her program daily as shown by her health and strength.

One day during class, a student interrupted, "Excuse me. I'd like to say something. I have been to the Boston retreat where I was taught by Dr. Ann.

"One day while slowly trudging up the second flight of steps to the fourth floor of the big manse, I heard, 'Excuse me!'

"I turned around to see Dr. Ann with a large box in her arms extended out fully in front of her loaded with heavy books. As I stepped aside, she zipped past me up the stairs all the way to the fourth floor with those heavy books!"

The lady added incredulously, "I could not have packed that load *down one* flight of steps - let alone up four flights."

Perhaps as food enzymes are broken apart in the stomach, the light energy stored in raw foods is released to do its healing work. But whatever it is, more research needs to be conducted to determine this healing life force in raw and living foods.

It is like putting money in savings to build up a depleted bank account. With raw and living foods the body's life force renews and addresses other important processes such as healing, strengthening, and regeneration.

Chapter 4
Ode to Green Foods

Spring is the time of year when daffodils, redbuds, and dogwoods blossom, and trees and grasses turn green once again. After braving the elements through the frigid, bleak winter, our ancestors took advantage of the bounties of spring. They dug up sassafras and other roots for making cleansing teas to "clear out and thin the blood." Dark leafy greens were welcomed as the first fresh food in spring after the stored food from winter had shriveled and started rotting.

As soon as the greens came up, my grandmother foraged for poke, narrow dock, wild mustard, dandelion, lamb's quarters, and many others for the family meal that day. She also collected all the greens she could find out of the fields, carefully washed them, and stuffed as many as she could get into a quart jar. Then she filled the jars with water and some salt before setting them outdoors in a tub of water over a fire to be boiled and sealed for what was called "copack" in those days. In this way, she provided for her family's supply of greens for the upcoming winter months.

Today we know that foods from all colors of the plant kingdom provide a full spectrum of nutrition, antioxidants, and many healthful phytochemicals, both known and unknown to science, but the many healing properties of leafy green foods seem to get little attention. I simply cannot write this book without extolling the virtues of raw leafy greens and grasses, of which the health benefits are not found in any other food.

Raw greens offer a rich source of vitamins, alkalizing minerals, phytonutrients, and antioxidants all in one package and are probably the most nutritious food on the earth. Dr. Ed Davis maintains that there is far more nutrition in a meadow of grasses than there is in a banquet table heavily weighed with food (1).

Raw greens are very alkalizing, and the body does not become sick in an alkaline state (2). The blood must be a pH of 7.35 to 7.45 for the body to perform optimally (3). When the blood pH dips lower, the blood draws alkalizing minerals from various parts of the body to re-establish a favorable (higher) pH and restore proper alkalinity. With time, acidic blood leeches calcium, magnesium, and other alkalizing minerals out of areas of the body such as the bones, predisposing the body to osteoporosis and other diseases. However, raw greens restore proper blood pH.

Raw greens also alkalize the oral cavity. According to Davis, who works with the pH of the body in his practice, the pH of the liver and mouth are the same and ideally should be 6.4 (4). It is when the pH of the mouth becomes lower that we start craving acidic foods such as meat, dairy, or pseudo-foods. As we eat acidic foods, the body becomes acidic, making a perfect climate for illness and disease. Raw greens, however, work to restore proper pH in the mouth and gastrointestinal tract for good digestion.

Raw greens and grasses are highly energizing. Magnesium, iron, B vitamins, and other nutrients in greens are vital for the cells to convert carbohydrates into energy. Raw leafy greens and grasses are probably the richest source of these nutrients. This is one reason why over time an ounce or two of fresh squeezed wheatgrass juice energizes the body until only a few hours of sleep are required each night. Wigmore awakened in the wee hours of the morning to research and write until she stopped to teach her program to students during the day with only a few hours of sleep each night from the light energy of green foods.

There is something about green foods that fortifies the pancreas which produces insulin and stabilizes blood sugar levels in the body. On client intake forms, I consistently see it across the board. When clients start their day with carbohydrates such as cereal, toast, rolls, donuts, even a healthy fruit smoothie, then later in the day they eat refined, processed sugars, such as cookies or candy. But when I put them on a salad with dark leafy greens, freshly squeezed green juices or smoothies, or wheatgrass juice for breakfast, their bodies become fortified, and they do not eat foods with refined sugars later in the day. Instead, they feel more satisfied, no longer craving addictive foods. Sugary foods become too rich and are shunned.

There are a number of anecdotal reports from both type 1 and type 2 diabetics whose blood sugar levels stabilized simply by consuming green smoothies made of raw organic blended fruit, greens, and water (5). A study in Spain indicates that the phytanic acid in the chlorophyll of greens may be useful in the treatment of type 2 diabetes (6). Another factor in leafy greens may be their rich source of magnesium. Magnesium deficiency has been linked to type 2 diabetes (7,8), and with over 65% of Americans deficient in magnesium (9), is it any wonder that 26 million Americans are diabetic with 79 million estimated to be pre-diabetic (10)?

There is still another property in greens not found in other foods that is important for good health. It is the green coloring pigment known as chlorophyll that provides the most important of all nutrients for both plants and animals - oxygen. Oxygen is required for all life to grow and flourish on Earth. Indeed, without green plants, there would be no life at all on this planet (11).

So why is chlorophyll so powerfully life-sustaining for the body? Found in leafy greens, chlorophyll is probably the best source created by Nature for cleansing and oxygenating the blood as well as restoring blood pH. The chlorophyll molecule is very similar to the hemoglobin molecule in red blood cells (12). Each hemoglobin molecule packs four molecules of oxygen. And just like hemoglobin, each chlorophyll molecule packs four molecules of oxygen. But instead of iron in its center as in hemoglobin, chlorophyll holds magnesium (see figure A).

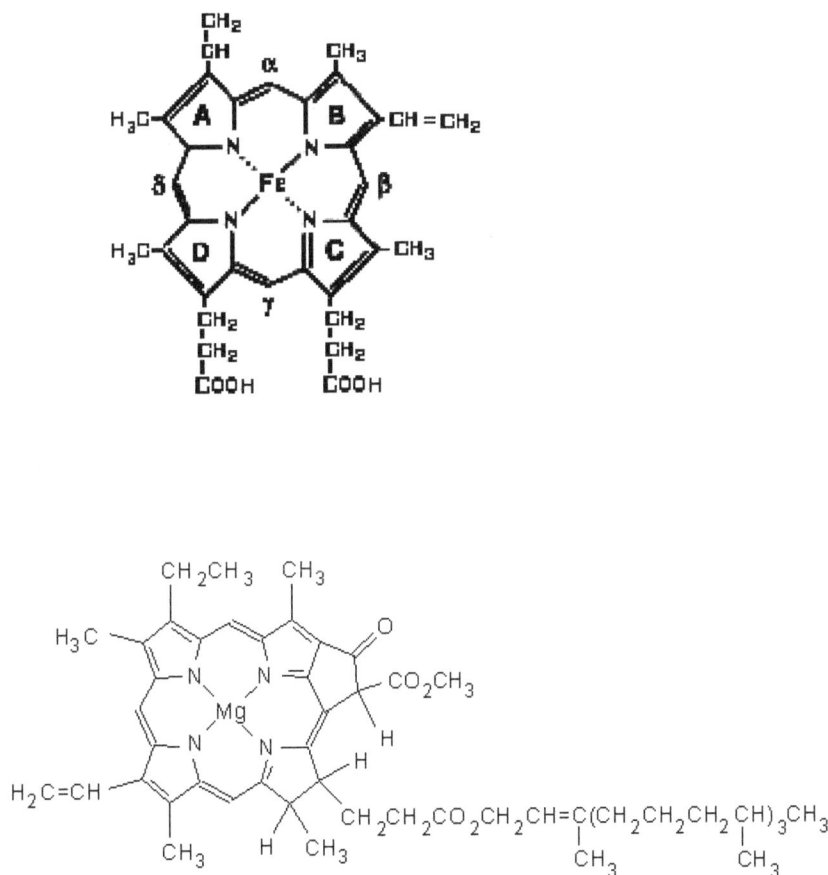

Figure A: Molecular Structure of hemoglobin (top) and chlorophyll (bottom).

Perhaps the iron found in green foods such as spinach replaces the magnesium in chlorophyll to manufacture more hemoglobin and red blood cells. But to be certain - chlorophyll increases oxygen in the blood to be distributed throughout the body.

Chlorophyll deodorizes the body (13). It fights infection by building up the body's defense mechanism and protects white blood cells of the immune system from DNA damage (14). It is highly effective in cases of chronic pancreatitis (15) and foodborne illness (16). Its antioxidant properties protect the body from radiation (17), and chlorophyll breaks down cancer cells (18).

Among many things that break down optimal numbers of healthy red blood cells are fungal pathogens, which rob the cells of iron and cause the cells to merge into a formless, dysfunctional clump (19). Another is stress, which causes red blood cells to clump together, making it more difficult to pack oxygen. Iron counts and the manufacture of new red blood cells are reduced (20,21). The heart then has to pump that much harder to deliver more oxygen, which decreases energy levels until life may seem overwhelming.

Sugar has been found to reduce white blood cells, which are the body's line of defense against foreign invaders that cause disease. One teaspoon of sugar can turn off the body's disease-fighting cells for up to five hours (22). Considering that sugar is such a staple in today's diet, is it any wonder that diseases continue to skyrocket?

People can only be as healthy as their blood is clean and healthy. They must have blood with a healthy pH free of harmful microorganisms, parasites, and toxins; plenty of white blood cells to fight toxic invaders; and many unclumped red blood cells distributing lots of healing oxygen throughout the body. As the body's toxic load lightens, energy levels increase, and thinking becomes clear and focused. One wakes up earlier of a morning, and the days become longer with more time in the evening for unwinding and relaxing.

Still yet, greens have an even greater purpose on this earth. Greens not only cleanse, feed, and heal the body - they also cleanse, feed, and heal the Earth. During photosynthesis, greens feed on sunshine, water, and carbon dioxide given off by animals and mankind and give off carbohydrates and oxygen to feed animals and mankind. When this cycle between the animal and plant kingdoms is balanced, the Earth heals and restores.

Nature also uses leaves on trees to filter particulate matter and pollutants from the air we breathe (23). Grasses are powerfully cleansing, too. A field of wheatgrass dramatically cleanses and refreshes the air.

Green leaves and grasses also provide sinkholes for carbon dioxide to be soaked up from the atmosphere to fight global warming. It is unlikely that global warming will cease until mankind replaces concrete and pavement with forests to help restore the ecological balance required by Nature to support life on Mother Earth as we know it today.

Greens are the only source in which all of these properties can be found in one food. While leafy greens may be the least of our favorite foods, they are a vital part of our diet. All life stems from green foods. They are the basis of the food chain from the whale that eats the fish that eats the algae and plankton (green sea vegetables) to the man and woman who eat the fish, cow, and deer that thrive on algae, green grasses, and leaves.

Stop and think - if the horse, cow, and deer can grow big and strong simply by eating and chewing on nothing more than grass all day long day after day, then how beneficial dark leafy greens must be for good health. Certainly more research needs to be conducted to determine the healing powers of green foods for the healing of Earth as well as mankind.

Linda Lamar Ruff, R.D.

Chapter 5
Raw Juices for Healing

He was sixty-one years old and in seemingly good health when he became hospitalized. His diagnosis was diverticulitis with microperforation. In other words, his colon had an inflamed outpouching with a "pinhole." The doctor and surgeon at the hospital recommended surgery, but he did not "want anyone cutting" on him.

Once he was released from the hospital, he consulted with a doctor who put him on a three-day juice fast along with my support and instruction on the proper diet to keep his colon healthy. After the fast, I put him on raw and living foods. Three months later not only were his symptoms gone, but he was surprised to find that the pain in his back that he had endured for two years had disappeared.

Juicing is becoming increasingly popular for its healing powers, and raw juice bars can be found in many cities across the nation. So what is juicing?

It consists of freshly-squeezed juices mechanically extracted from the pulp (fiber) of raw fruits and vegetables. Raw juices provide a concentrated source of enzymes, the life force within the food. When the body's energy levels and life forces are low, the enzymes in raw juices reactivate the body processes and renew the life force within. Since the enzymes become sluggish and start dying at temperatures above 110 degrees Fahrenheit, the fruits and vegetables used for juicing cannot be cooked, pasteurized, or irradiated.

Unlike water during a fast, raw juices contain concentrated amounts of vitamins, alkalizing minerals, antioxidants, phytochemicals, and countless other nutrients that stabilize blood sugar levels and provide optimal energy. So energized was the above gentleman that he actually worked third shift every night during his three-day fast.

The healthy benefits of pure raw fruit and vegetable juices are much overlooked. Juices are good for fighting bacteria (1), and fresh lemon juice fights cholera without harm to the body (2). Juicing has been found to reduce the risk of cardiovascular disease (3), and a study in Texas found that two cups of raw carrot juice on a daily basis lowered systolic blood pressure (4). Raw juices have been found to protect genes from toxicity (5), and cabbage and sauerkraut juices have shown to prevent cancer (6).

Raw juices are also loaded with a plethora of antioxidants, which restore health and "youth" the body. When the body is not in a healthy state, cells prematurely decompose and release many unstable free radicals which attach to other compounds in the body and create further damage. The antioxidants in raw juices, however, stabilize free radicals to fight degeneration and aging of the body. The above Texas study found that the raw carrot juice increased antioxidant levels (7), which protect against cancer and increase lifespan (8). When consuming fresh raw juices on a daily basis, people are amazed by how much younger they feel and look.

Raw juices provide concentrated nourishment that is far more quickly and easily absorbed into the body than eating foods at a meal. While it may take hours before a meal is fully digested from a healthy gastrointestinal tract and fully absorbed into the bloodstream, it takes only minutes for the juices to be absorbed and distributed where needed for healing and maintenance. This is critical for someone with a life-threatening illness.

Raw juices fight constipation by stimulating peristalsis, the wave-like motion that pushes food through the gastrointestinal tract and wastes out of the body. Instead of feeling bloated, raw juices leave one feeling full and satisfied. Raw juices also supply an excellent source of organic water, the second most important nutrient for the body. The live organic water in raw juices soaks up old matter in the gut and, with peristalsis, flushes debris and toxins out of the body. Better yet, raw juices clear out rubbish higher up in the gastrointestinal tract where colon cleansing cannot reach. Once the rubbish is cleared out of the way, raw juices hydrate the body and give the skin a soft, dewy glow. The juices not only flushed out the above gentleman's colon but also speeded the healing of diverticulitis.

Many might maintain that we can get the same nutrition by eating fruits and vegetables. However, getting the same amount of nutrients found in a glass of raw juice would require long hours of chewing several times the amount of produce. What's more, our foods are not as nutritional as they were sixty or more years ago. Sadly, it seems the agricultural industry has become more concerned with higher yields of crops than nutrition (9,10).

Is it any wonder that dinner plates are now larger than they were 100 years ago with obesity rampant? Is it any wonder that the latest nutritional guidelines now recommend 9-13 servings per day of fruits and vegetables, up from the former recommended 5-9 servings?

It is no wonder that substance abuse and addictions abound in many guises. When the body lacks the nutrient(s) required to function, it will crave and seek out that nutrient(s) until it satisfies that need. Juices from non-genetically engineered, local, raw organic produce with concentrated nutrition, antioxidants, and countless phytochemicals provide an excellent means of putting desperately needed nourishment into our bodies faster than the healthiest of foods can.

So what kind of juices did I provide the gentleman? Vegetable juices of carrots, beets, celery, and dark leafy greens; fruit smoothies; and sesame milkshakes with the pulp. The doctor said it was okay to include the pulp despite the microperforation. (For the recipes check out chapter 13.)

Juicing has been used for other health issues such as colds, hay fever, headaches, arthritis, and the list goes on. And it need not stop with humans. I have talked to people who have brought dying animals back to life simply by using healing wheatgrass juice.

While raw juices are a powerful cleanser, immune booster, and healer of the body, it is advisable to undertake a juice fast with the guidance of a health care practitioner experienced in fasting. On the other hand, a large glass of raw juice every day for breakfast or as a snack will certainly go a long way to promote good health.

Chapter 6
The Many Uses of Wheatgrass Juice

After leading an illustrious life as a soprano singer, she faded from the music scene due to ill health. Multiple sclerosis had left her bedridden with nothing to look forward to except the final day when she would pass on.

At the same time in another part of Boston, there was a concert pianist who had dropped out of the musical arena with emphysema. With each passing day he fought to breathe, anticipating the final end to be a just few months.

And only blocks from the concert pianist was a basso with painfully swollen joints from arthritis. Seemingly, the only relief was death.

Meanwhile an "angel of mercy" in the form of Ann Wigmore had established a route where she delivered fresh-squeezed wheatgrass juice to many, including the three musical professionals.

A few weeks later, along with an evening meal of vegetables, the basso with arthritis hobbled outside into the sunshine where he amazed acquaintances.

A month later the soprano with multiple sclerosis was walking short distances and visiting the beauty salon, where she had not been for years.

A few months later the concert pianist with emphysema could walk without assistance.

Through Wigmore, the three joyfully rediscovered each other after seven years. So happy were they to be productive once again that they devoted the rest of their lives to helping others (1).

The first time I attended the Ann Wigmore Natural Health Institute in Puerto Rico, I saw people not only drinking wheatgrass juice but putting it on their skin, in their eyes, and up their noses. I said to myself, "These people are obsessed with wheatgrass juice!"

But make no mistake about it. Despite its looks or taste, more people are going to wheatgrass juice for concentrated nutrition and healing. When grown in clean, rich soil, wheatgrass juice is not only a superior source of nutrition but also a powerful cleanser for the body.

Chlorophyll (the green pigment in plants), which is in all grasses, is so important that all life on Earth cannot exist without it. Since the rays of the sun are stored as energy in chlorophyll, everyone derives energy from the sun whether we consume green grass, or we get it second-hand by eating the cow that eats the green grass or the fish that eats green seaweed. However, getting energy first-hand from chlorophyll-rich green grass provides far more strength and endurance than getting it second-hand through meat or fish.

The chlorophyll in wheatgrass juice rebuilds the bloodstream. In India there were anecdotal reports of patients with thalassemia (a form of anemia) reducing blood transfusion amounts by drinking wheatgrass juice. Therefore, a study was conducted which found blood transfusion amounts were reduced by up to 40% with no side effects (2).

Interestingly, another study found that while there were no side effects, wheat grass treatment did not reduce the amount of transfusion (3). The difference? The study with no results incorporated wheatgrass *tablets* while the study that reduced transfusion amounts used fresh-squeezed wheatgrass juice grown at home by families of the patients.

Another study in India found wheatgrass juice lowered triglycerides and total cholesterol in rats with high cholesterol (4).

Wheatgrass juice aids digestive healing. Anecdotal reports of wheatgrass juice in the treatment of gastrointestinal disorders prompted a study in Israel (5). The study found wheatgrass juice safely reduced rectal bleeding and improved ulcerative colitis.

In Malaysia wheatgrass has been found to break down cancer cells in leukemia (6), and in Israel the juice was shown to reduce dosage and improve effectiveness of chemotherapy (7).

At the Institute wheatgrass juice was a large part of the program which successfully treated many conditions. While many grasses have powerful healing properties, Wigmore chose to use wheatgrass because when grown in rich organic soil, it comes closest to meeting man's nutritional needs.

Wheatgrass juice strengthens the pancreas, thus improving the blood sugar levels of the students. It bypasses the gastrointestinal tract for faster delivery into the bloodstream, which gives an ailing digestive tract a chance to rest and heal. This can mean the difference of life or death to an individual with just a short time to live.

Wigmore felt that the high oxygen content of chlorophyll-rich wheatgrass dissolves scars in the lungs from breathing acid gases and halts the growth of unfriendly bacteria, infections, and cancer cells that create odor. As a deodorizer, wheatgrass eliminates garlic odor, bad breath, perspiration, menstrual odors, and urine and fecal smells.

Wheatgrass juice has been used for tooth decay. When the pulp is held in the mouth for several minutes, the juice fights infection in the gums, eliminating gingivitis and pyorrhea. It also works as a gargle for sore throat.

Wheatgrass juice is great for skin disorders, including eczema and psoriasis. It heals sores and wounds and speeds skin grafting. With improved diet, it will eliminate acne and remove scars after seven or eight months.

This is the reason I saw green people walking around the Institute coated with wheatgrass juice. They used the juice to pull impurities out of the skin in exchange for a smooth, glowing complexion. Within weeks of this treatment, I saw actors and models go back to their agencies with the skin of a celebrity. One lady applied the pulp of wheatgrass along with some herbs onto melanoma on her arm. By the end of the day, her skin cancer was reduced in size.

The high enzyme and magnesium content in wheatgrass helps to restore sex hormones and fertility. Many a woman who could never conceive has found herself pregnant after following the Living Foods Lifestyle® at the Institute.

Wheatgrass juice even restores natural hair color. Over a period of several months Wigmore watched her hair turn from gray back to its original brown.

To get the most benefits from wheatgrass juice, it should be freshly squeezed and immediately taken on an empty stomach upon arising first thing in the morning. Then wait twenty to thirty minutes before eating so that the body will quickly absorb it. It immediately goes to work where it is needed.

When first starting out on a wheatgrass regime, drink only one or two ounces one to two times a day. As the body's toxic load reduces, an individual will alkalize and develop a tolerance for more. Then one can gradually increase the amount.

Never drink over six ounces at one time. Too much wheatgrass juice can free up toxins faster than the body can throw them off, and one will become sick with the backlogged toxins. Also know that as much as eight or ten ounces of the juice throughout the day can leave one wide awake at night until the wee hours of the morning – so highly energizing is this potent elixir.

Occasionally, a student with gluten intolerance and sensitivities would come who was concerned about drinking the wheatgrass juice.

Yet not a one of the countless students with gluten intolerance and sensitivities who came through the doors of the Institute ever had problems with wheatgrass juice. The heavy proteins which trigger symptoms are found in the berries and not the grass itself.

Unfortunately, not everyone easily tolerates wheatgrass juice at first. This is because their bodies are acidic from toxins. Some people are so toxic that the second they swallow the juice, their gag reflex is instantly activated. This is because the juice is doing its job. It immediately sucks out the toxins upon contact and comes back up via regurgitation. But with time as the body detoxifies, it becomes more alkaline and accepts the alkaline juice and greens much easier.

There is yet another avenue of incorporating the cleansing and healing powers of wheatgrass juice. At the Institute, following an enema or colon hydrotherapy, a rectal implant of wheatgrass juice was used to cleanse, heal, and tone the colon. The implant eliminates constipation while pulling impurities out of the liver, such as heavy metals, drug deposits, parasites, and other toxins.

To incorporate a rectal implant, immediately after clearing out the colon, lie on a slant board or surface on the left side of the body, preferably with the head lower than the buttocks. Simply squeeze with a syringe bulb approximately six ounces of fresh wheatgrass juice into the rectum and hold it. After five minutes, roll onto the back for another fifteen minutes. Hold the implant for a total of twenty minutes, if possible. After twenty minutes, simply release the contents from the rectum into the stool.

This may seem arduous the first few times, but once the colon clears out, it becomes easier to retain the juice rectally. Once the channels in the colon are open, the juice is immediately absorbed into the liver, pancreas, and other areas of the body where it is needed for cleansing and healing. It is at this point that it may not be necessary to lie with the implant elevated any more than five minutes. With time the colon becomes so clean that one may be able to hold the implant without having to release it.

I could tell of more stories and healings, but need I say more? Of all those touted as superfoods, wheatgrass juice is the most powerful and healing of all foods on this planet. When taking wheatgrass juice on a daily basis, hunger, fatigue, and addictions are replaced with good energy, endurance, and vitality. When is the last time that you felt so satisfied with your meal that you pushed your plate of food away? It is a peaceful way to live.

Chapter 7
Sprouts and Nutrition

She found the monkey in a pet show. Because it was sick, she purchased "the poor creature" for a small amount.

Since the lady had been eating nourishing seeds for her health, she fed them to little "Precious," but Precious was having difficulty eating them. It was then that the lady noticed that each tooth had been extracted to keep Precious from biting and defending herself.

The lady then softened the seeds by soaking them in water and placing them between damp towels. Lo and behold! after a few days the seeds sprouted. As she fed Precious the sprouted seeds, the health of the monkey returned, and together they lived many years thereafter (1).

That lady was Dr. Ann Wigmore, and this is how we have come to know sprouting. Thanks to Dr. Ann, nearly sixty years later the word "sprouts" has become a common household term around the world.

So what about sprouts restored the health of Precious? For one thing, the sprouting process predigests the protein into amino acids, fats into fatty acids, and carbohydrates into simple sugars, which makes digestion easier - a boon for individuals with digestive disturbances.

What's more, sprouts have exponentially higher amounts of nutrition than the mature plant that it later becomes. Sprouts are the babies of the plant kingdom where all plants start. The broccoli stalk grows from the tiny little sprouted broccoli seed. The apple tree grows from a sprouted seed to produce apples. Even the lowly blade of wheatgrass begins as a sprouted wheat berry.

In the animal kingdom, during gestation, if the mother does not have enough nutrition in her body to support both her and the developing fetus, then the fetus gets the mother's nutrition for a good healthy start in life. It is the same in the plant kingdom - baby sprouts get more nutrition than the mature plant.

A study in Spain found that germination raised the content of the amino acid lysine in beans, peas, and lentils compared with unsprouted seeds (2). According to the research of Wigmore, bean and sunflower sprouts have more protein than beef, chicken, and fish (3), and very small amounts of protein, vitamins, and other nutrients in raw seeds increase exponentially when those same seeds are sprouted (4).

Antioxidants are also higher in sprouts than in mature vegetables (5). But that's not all! Sprouts are rich in enzymes, the vital life force which is missing in cooked and processed pseudofoods. Sprouted broccoli seeds increase coenzyme Q_{10} content, which improves cholesterol function and protects the heart (6,7). Small quantities in sprouted form are shown to be rich with detoxifying enzymes that protect from bladder cancer and cancers caused by chemicals just as effectively as the mature broccoli plant does (8,9).

Green buckwheat sprouts fight inflammation in colon cancer (10), and both broccoli and fenugreek sprouts have properties that fight infection in peptic ulcers and gastritis (11,12).

This is why squirrels busy themselves burying nuts in the fall. The nut lies dormant in the ground until the soil becomes wet enough from rains to soak and sprout the nut. Then the squirrel digs up and eats the sprouted nut for sustenance during the cold winter months (13).

But before the seeds can sprout, they must be soaked in clean filtered water to release enzyme inhibitors. Mother Nature uses enzyme inhibitors to keep seeds from sprouting and to protect the seed and its nutrients from being lost until the conditions are right for the seed to grow and mature into a plant. Then the nutrients and enzymes are easily bioavailable for the body.

Unfortunately, the risks of foodborne illness from eating sprouts get far more attention than the nutritional and healing benefits of sprouts. But unknown to most people, foodborne illness does not originate with sprouts, onions, spinach, cantaloupe, or any other plant source. Foodborne pathogens stem from the fecal matter of animals, and the manure and waste runoff from the livestock industry and factory farming have become a major problem. Waste runoff has been shown to contaminate water supplies that are used to fertilize and irrigate fields. The lack of toilet facilities for field workers creates food hazards. Also, improper handling and refrigeration during storage and shipping to stores and restaurants further increase risk of contamination.

However, sprouts are grown and eaten on a daily basis at the Ann Wigmore Natural Health Institute. As evidenced by countless students who have experienced countless healings, the benefits of eating sprouts far outweigh the risks, and an outbreak of foodborne illness at the Institute has never been a problem.

So where to find sprouts? They may be found in the produce section in supermarkets and on salad bars and sandwiches in restaurants and delicatessens. But the best and safest way to eat sprouts is to grow them fresh in your own home. It costs only pennies per day, and it is so easy!

But first, for precautionary measures against foodborne illness, many follow this process before eating raw produce and sprouting seeds. Simply mix a solution of several drops of food grade hydrogen peroxide with enough water to fill a spray bottle. Then spray seeds and produce and let set. The bubbling action indicates that the hydrogen peroxide is destroying bacteria and other microorganisms that are on the seeds and produce. After several minutes, rinse the seeds with cold water.

Another method is to add ten or twelve drops of grapefruit seed extract oil to a pan of water and set seeds and produce in the pan. After several minutes, rinse the seeds with cold water. Both of these methods effectively remove any pathogenic microorganisms while leaving nutritional benefits intact.

Next, simply cover the bottom of a gallon or half-gallon jar with sprout seeds found at health food or specialty stores. Secure the top of the jar with a screen lid or mesh fabric held in place with a rubber band. Then cover and soak one part seeds to two parts pure filtered water to release the enzyme inhibitors so that the seeds can sprout.

Small seeds, such as alfalfa or radish, may soak for four hours while larger seeds, such as chickpeas, may soak eight to ten hours or overnight. The seeds will swell to approximately double their size.

When finished soaking, pour off the water and tip the jar sideways to rest in a rack and drain. Make certain to leave enough room in the opening of the jar to allow for air to get to the seeds to keep them from souring. Rinse and drain twice a day until tails or "sprouts" grow for as long as you want them.

And there you have it! Sprouts can be eaten in salads and sandwiches and added to raw smoothies and soups.

So have some fun and try sprouting. Your body will appreciate it.

And the next time you see sprouts in a restaurant or store, think of Dr. Ann Wigmore and little Precious. It is because of them that you and I know of sprouts today.

Chapter 8
Detoxification - The Right Hand of Living Foods

The food supply of today is not the same as that of our forefathers one hundred years ago. Breads were made fresh at home from the oven or a local baker from non-refined, non-genetically modified whole grains rich with fiber freshly ground from a neighboring mill. Pasture-fed cows were milked by hand each morning and evening for the day's fresh supply. Produce came straight from the garden fertilized with fresh farm manure that was turned into the soil. Fruit came from trees in the yard or a nearby orchard pollinated by local bees. Meat from livestock raised at home or a nearby farm was butchered at home or by the neighborhood butcher.

Sadly, not only has our food supply changed since then, but we are not as strong and healthy as our forefathers nor could we toil and labor as they did. Instead, our grains and produce have been commercially raised to withstand a bath of herbicides, pesticides, and insecticides that kill the soil and all other surrounding forms of life. Milk is heat-treated or pasteurized to last unrefrigerated for six or more months without spoiling. Livestock is inhumanely raised in factory farms with antibiotics and growth hormones which alter the body's metabolism. Since carcasses are currently going through the slaughterhouses at such a fast rate to keep up with demand, the USDA now allows meat to harbor fecal matter as long as it is invisible to the naked eye (1). Is it any wonder that foodborne illness and disease are becoming more prevalent?

Studies are showing that regardless of the working or living environment, all subjects carried chemicals, pollutants, and pesticides in their bodies - many of which were not in existence 75 years ago (2,3). Today my files are rampant with current research of how toxic chemicals and pollutants affect not only our health but our thought processes and emotions as well. Let's face it – as our environment and food supply are compromised and contaminated, so is our health.

What's worse, research shows that while food consumption is climbing, the nutritional profile of our food supply has declined dramatically compared to that of fifty years ago (4,5). Unfortunately, our foods are manufactured for eye appeal and years of shelf life without spoilage. Stop and think - if our foods do not break down on the shelf, then why should we think they will break down in our gut?

Any beneficial properties that may remain in the food have become so altered that the body no longer recognizes them, or else the foods do not provide the nutrients for the body to function properly in the first place. Thus, we feed our bodies false or pseudofoods.

Unfortunately, when the body is not fed the essential nutrients, peristalsis (which pushes food and residue through the body) cannot function, nor can the body manufacture the digestive flora and acids necessary to break down foods and assimilate any nutrients. The colon becomes overwhelmed with heavy fiberless pseudofoods which can accumulate and back up in the gut to create constipation. There the matter can become trapped and encrusted against the walls of the gastrointestinal tract, creating further constipation, diverticulosis, and other colon disorders. Passage of nutrients, such as large molecules of vitamins and proteins, becomes difficult through this barrier, which sets up a nutrient-deficient body for addictions (6,7,8).

The encrusted colon may then expand like a balloon and press against organs in the body, making it hard for them to function. The swollen colon will weigh down on the bladder causing it to hold less urine. Then one has to release more often, making more bathroom trips necessary (9). As more nutritionally depleted food enters the nutrient-starved body, the rubbish gets pushed aside and heaped into weaker parts of the colon and body along with trapped fluids. With time the rubbish and fluids can grow into a human landfill, creating an enlarged abdominal area and excess weight, thus providing a happy home where molds and fungus, parasites, and harmful bacteria and microorganisms breed and give off offending wastes and by-products. Coupled with the undigested matter, fermentation and putrefaction create gas, bloating, and abdominal discomfort. As a result, dead pseudofoods can create obesity that masks starvation (10).

Raw and living foods, however, are extremely powerful for healing from these health disorders, but it is only half of the process. The other half is body cleansing. One can get the best of clean foods loaded with powerful nutrition, antioxidants, enzymes, and other healing phytochemicals, but if the body is backlogged with dirt and toxins, then the best of foods only becomes more added toxins that the body cannot use (11). Therefore, body cleansing is the right hand of raw and living foods; one cannot work without the other, and healing cannot occur until the bowel is clean.

There are many signs of toxicity in the body. Some signs are feeling tired, lethargic, and drowsy after a meal instead of energized. At other times without explanation one may sometimes feel overwhelmed with fatigue and simply cannot move.

Sprayed chemicals that travel through the air may cause an individual to suddenly feel overwhelmed with weakness or sleep for no apparent reason. When this happens, the body draws from all of its physical, mental, and productive energies just to throw off the toxins.

Anytime there is a burning sensation deep within the body, poisonous chemicals may be at work. If the hands or feet itch where scratching will not relieve it, there may be toxins deep inside. When the rectum burns during a bowel movement or colon hydrotherapy, the body may be releasing poisons.

If the throat needs clearing when speaking, this may be a sign that what has been eaten is not digesting and moving through the system very efficiently. Instead, the undigested matter may be backing up to the throat and getting in the way when speaking.

If the vision seems dim or cloudy instead of crystal clear, or the print seems too small to read, the eyes may be storing dirt that hinders vision. When vision dims, sinuses become congested, the throat clogs, and hearing becomes faint and garbled, the head may be loaded with toxins. When one has trouble remembering, thinking clearly, or getting out the right words, toxins and heavy metals could be blocking neurotransmitters in the brain. When logic or reasoning becomes impaired, behavior can become irrational.

These symptoms are only a few clues that the body may be loaded with toxins which can breed disease and dying. I cannot emphasize enough the importance of a good detoxification program.

But how to go about it? Methods of detoxification ranging from herbs to fasting to enemas have been around for centuries. Today many products are available for cleansing the colon and body of heavy metals, yeast and fungal infections, parasites, and other toxins.

But before I discuss any methods, I must emphasize – before undertaking any cleansing program, it is best to consult with a health professional experienced in body cleansing. Depending upon the health of the individual, many questions and complications can arise, and it is best to have guidance from someone who can provide qualified support.

There are two major methods of detoxification – fasting and colon cleansing. Fasting is an effective time-honored method practiced further back than Biblical times. When fasting, one abstains from foods while imbibing only liquids for a period of one or more days. Once the body adapts to this practice, the digestive tract enjoys its rest from its labors and cleanses while the cells of the body shed toxins at an increased pace (12).

There are two different kinds of fasts - water and juice. During water fasts, only water is consumed. Copious amounts of clean filtered water clear unwanted debris from the colon and kidneys and rehydrate the body.

On the other hand, juice fasting is done with fresh-squeezed juices mechanically extracted from unpasteurized, non-genetically modified, organic raw produce, which provides water in a live alkaline form. While juices made from fruits (such as apples) and from root vegetables (such as carrots) are high in sugar, adding celery and dark leafy greens balances out the sugars so that during the fast, one feels full and satisfied without food cravings. Many with a short time to live have reduced or eliminated cancer and other illnesses with fasts on raw juices while maintaining good energy levels and health. During the first week at the Institute, a three-day period of juices and pureed foods was used to initiate the detoxification period. Then on the first day after the three day cleanse, light raw foods were introduced back into the meals to re-acclimate students to whole foods.

The other major method of detoxification is colon flushing, which research shows to be safe and effective (13,14). At the Institute enemas and colon hydrotherapy are used as part of the Living Foods Lifestyle®.

At the Institute I have seen those who chose to eat the living foods while foregoing colon cleansing. In a matter of days as the bloodstream carried dirt and rubbish from the cells to the colon, the colon could not clear out the collected matter fast enough. Consequently, the student became ill. Therefore, the colon needs to be clear and free flowing so that backlogged toxins can be freely released.

More clinics and health retreats around the world are providing these services in a professional setting with health care practitioners certified in colon hydrotherapy. Technology also provides open-system equipment for those familiar with the procedure and desiring to cleanse in the privacy of their home.

There are advantages, however, of going to a professional hydrotherapist who uses a closed system. A good professional will massage the colon and other areas of the body which stimulates the release of matter, leaving one feeling clean and fresh at the end. Also an experienced hydrotherapist will discover when medical services are needed and refer the client to a medical professional. He or she may also refuse to provide service when colonics are contraindicated and instead send the client to a medical professional. Always consult with one experienced in these matters who can offer wise counsel during colon cleansing.

Once the colon is free of matter, both it and the body can slowly regain their normal shape (15). And unlike cooked and pseudofoods, the gut assimilates the concentrated nutrition found in raw and living foods very efficiently, for all bloating and gas totally disappear on the Living Foods Lifestyle®.

For the best results, fasting one day a week on clean water, rejuvelac (when indicated), and raw juices go hand-in-hand with a colon flush in the evening. This allows time for the digestive tract to rest and clear out rubbish while each cell in the body "cleans house" and sweeps the dirt out into the bloodstream. At the end of the day, after the digestive tract and bloodstream have carried away and deposited wastes in the colon, bathing the colon flushes those wastes away. Following a colon flush, a rectal implant of wheatgrass juice is strongly recommended to suck out matter reluctant to leave its happy home. Many a colon hydrotherapist has been astonished to see the amount of matter the wheatgrass juice pulls out of a "clean" colon that was thought to be empty. As stated in chapter 6, a wheatgrass juice implant also pulls impurities out of the liver and other organs where a colon flush does not reach.

No food should be eaten until the next morning when the previous day's fast is broken with a *break-fast* of light raw foods. This process may continue once a day every week until the body is thoroughly clean. With time the results are extremely rewarding as good health is restored and the "youthing" process of the body is reactivated.

Sadly, our planet is getting so dirty and toxic that detoxification should be done periodically. While detoxification is *very* important, it is not easy. It requires much work, discipline, and perseverance over a long period of time as the cleansing and healing process may take months, even years (16). After all, our body's natural biorhythms and cells function at a much slower rate than the hectic pace of today's society.

When embarking on a raw and living foods program, the body generally takes three to four days to adjust. But once it adapts, it runs forward with the new lifestyle. As the body becomes more alkaline, people's tastes change. No longer do they crave the acidic pseudo-foods and drinks that once controlled their lives. Instead they become surprised to find themselves wanting clean, healthy foods that were formerly disliked, and those greens that seemed so bitter now taste sweet.

Other unexpected changes occur, such as the disappearance of chronic aches and pains. Inches melt from the middle, and wrinkles diminish or disappear to create a smoother, glowing complexion. As one removes wastes from the colon, along with a totally raw lifestyle, one finds that instead of degenerating or aging, the body actually regenerates and becomes younger.

While this period was difficult to follow, by the end of the week the students felt a transformation in themselves and also saw it in others. They experienced the joy that comes with healing and a deeper spirituality that comes with living in the higher dimension of the Living Foods Lifestyle®. It was such a delight to discover the hidden beauty of the students once they shed their baggage.

But do keep in mind - the cleansing and healing processes will continue indefinitely while one lives totally on raw and living foods. But once one reintroduces cooked foods back into the body, the healing processes slow down dramatically - if not stop. At the Institute I saw students who went out for cooked foods only to later regret not following the program when they saw the life and healing in others.

Chapter 9
Deeper Cleansing

While working in the office one day, a gentleman made reservations for himself and his wife. He also insisted on scheduling daily colonic appointments for each of them. Since the Institute only provided for three a week per person, I kept informing him I could not do that. Yet he kept insisting that he and his wife should get one each day to which I calmly replied it was not possible. He continued to insist, and I continued to calmly state I could not do that.

After great length, he finally asked of me, "Okay, then. Will you please contact the colonic therapist and ask her for me?"

Grateful to become unstuck from our loop, I cheerfully responded, "Certainly, I can do that."

While the therapist did not give them one each day, she instructed me to schedule him and his wife each three a week. With that he became satisfied.

Many colon hydrotherapists state that ten to twelve sessions are all that is necessary to clear out the colon under average health conditions. Like the man above, many think that all they have to do is clean out the colon, and then they can go merrily on their way. But just because the colon is clean is no sign the body is clean. After all, the body's pace is not fast enough to clear out years of accumulated dirt and toxins in just a few short weeks. While a clean colon is necessary for detoxification, it is only the first step in the process. For once the colon becomes clean and regains its normal shape, it can back off other organs which frees them to clear out trapped toxins on a deeper molecular level. This is the next step in body cleansing.

Two important organs that need flushing are the two kidneys. If the colon is not free-flowing, then the rubbish and debris from the cells get shunted to the kidneys, creating an extra workload for them and causing toxic build-up and infections. Therefore, it is vital to drink no less than two quarts of clean, filtered water, fresh raw juices, and rejuvelac (when appropriate) to flush out the kidneys.

"Two quarts of water! How can I drink that much?" This is one response that I get.

Actually, it is simple. The body is thirstiest of a morning because very little water, if any, has been drunk throughout the night.

Therefore, it is easy to drink a quart immediately upon arising in the morning. The rest can be taken intermittently throughout the day.

Another response is, "I always bloat when I drink water."

Any bloating or swelling may indicate that fluids may not be moving through the body. When the digestive tract does not have enough flora or acid to digest food and pass it through the system, fluid may become trapped with backlogged matter. Colon flushing can wash away much trapped fluid, which will alleviate stress on the kidneys and ultimately eliminate bloating.

Potassium deficiency may be another indication. Potassium is required for peristalsis, the muscular contraction that pushes food matter through the digestive tract and flushes out excess fluid (1). Good sources of potassium are watery fruits and melons.

Watermelon with seeds is an excellent source of potassium, is alkalizing, and when eaten by itself, is very powerful for soaking up and pulling old matter out of the gastrointestinal tract. It too is an excellent cleanser of the kidneys, and the seeds are highly nourishing for the kidneys (2,3). Always eat watermelons with the seeds.

The white part of the melon next to the green rind is a valuable source of alkalizing minerals and nutrition (4). Many a time after eating watermelon did I carry the left-over rind to the ducks on the lake at my home only to watch them fight over the white part. Those ducks were smarter than me. They knew that the white rind of the melon holds far more concentrated nutrition than the sweet red part.

At the Institute watermelon, along with the white rind and heavily nutritious seeds, were juiced for breakfast during heavy detox days.

Still yet another response I get is, "When I drink water, I have to go to the bathroom all the time."

As stated in chapter 8, the enlarged colon can weigh down on the bladder, causing it to hold a smaller volume of fluid (5,6). But when doing a series of colon flushes, eventually the colon will clear out and lift up off the bladder. Then the bladder holds more urine, and one releases larger amounts far less often.

Once the colon and kidneys flow freely, other organs can "clean house" and release backlogged contents. But unlike the bowel and kidneys which protest loudly when they are overworked or diseased, the liver may work relentlessly for a lifetime before any chronic health condition is detected.

The liver has multitudes of duties. It regulates protein and carbohydrate metabolism, stores vitamins and minerals, manufactures hormones and enzymes, and filters harmful bacteria, chemicals, and toxins from the blood. The liver is the major fat burner of the body, and the constant influx of processed fatty pseudofoods and alcoholic beverages leads to a "fatty" or congested liver.

Signs of liver overload can be any of the following: poor digestion, acid reflux, or intolerance to fatty foods; blotchy red skin, rashes, or any skin disorder; "liver" or "age" spots, freckles, warts, and cherry angiomas (small red, raised spots); fluid retention, cellulite, or obesity; sinus issues, allergies, asthma, and respiratory illnesses; headaches and pain in the eyes and ears; poor hearing; blurred or clouded vision; "foggy" or clouded thinking; fatigue or hypoglycemia; yeast infection; cancer; parasites; and many ailments caused from backed up toxins waiting to be processed by the liver.

When the liver becomes overwhelmed, it dumps the excess in its storage area, the gallbladder. When an encrusted colon and small intestine squeeze against the ducts leading from the liver, gallbladder, and pancreas, the bile, hormones, insulin, and digestive enzymes cannot travel as efficiently through the ducts to the small intestine for digestion. With time harmful fats from meats, dairy, and pseudofoods can create excess weight, further squeezing against the liver, gallbladder, and other organs. Then the organs do not function as well and the overloaded liver, gallbladder, and ducts are at increased risk for gallstones (7).

Liver and gallbladder flushes can assist in the cleansing process. Many who have followed good health practices and done "the right things" throughout their lives are astounded to see what comes out of a liver flush.

While this was not part of the program at the Institute, a few took it upon themselves to do a liver flush. The naturopath who worked there, however, did *not* advise such a practice. She knew of one who tried to flush out her liver and gallbladder only to have a stone too large to pass become lodged in a duct. The individual then had to have the excruciatingly painful stone removed surgically. For this reason, the utmost of caution should be exercised under the guidance of a professional practitioner experienced in liver and gallbladder cleanses.

Another important system that works with the organs is the lymphatic system, which carries white blood cells that provide a defense mechanism against foreign material and pathogens that invade the body. Among other important functions, the spleen and lymph nodes filter wastes and chemicals from fats, which harbor environmental toxins. When the colon and liver are backlogged, toxic wastes back up into the lymph fluid and are carried and spread throughout the body (8,9).

A clean and optimally functioning lymphatic system is vital for a healthy immune system. With ongoing colon and liver flushes, the lymph system can drain its backlogged contents into the colon. Exercise is also very important in assisting this process. Brisk walking with vigorous swinging of the arms helps drain the lymph, and both skin brushing and jumping on a rebounder are excellent techniques that stimulate lymph movement through the body. Walking, skin brushing, and rebounding were part of the program at the Institute.

Once these organs are cleansed and functioning, toxic build-up can be removed from the skin, pancreas, lungs, heart, and other organs so that they can work efficiently.

The body cleanses from the inside out and the top down. But detoxification still may not be over. Last but not least, the top part of the body, the head, also needs cleansing. Toxic wastes in the brain can affect mental processes and how one feels (10,11,12).

When the colon, kidneys, liver, gallbladder, lymph system, and other organs start clearing out, the brain will start removing rubbish as well. The most effective and powerful way to assist the process is to snort wheatgrass juice up each nostril, as the young woman with mercury toxicity did in chapter 2. Simply lower the head back and with an eyedropper drip the juice into each nostril. As you keep the head back, feel the juice work its way down into the sinuses, behind the eyes, and into the brain. Once the rubbish starts coming out of the nose and mouth, one feels amazingly lighter and thinks clearer. Several flushes may be required before a full clearing of the head and sinuses is felt. As the head clears, the mind becomes sharp and focused, and remembering becomes much easier.

But during the cleansing process do be aware - unlike weighty cooked foods that keep our darker emotions stuffed and hidden, raw foods are light weight and allow the "ghosts and demons" that lurk deep within to drift up to the surface where we must face them. This is where emotional cleansing comes in.

Chapter 10
Emotional Cleansing

The pretty 29-year-old woman from North Carolina had undergone three days of heavy detoxification with liquid and pureed foods. It was nearly midnight when I listened to her as tears poured from her innermost being.

She and her former husband had abused drugs during their time together. When their little baby girl was born, the infant's digestive tract was not properly developed, so after a few months the infant died. Now without heavy cooked foods to sedate her grief and guilt, the lady was feeling responsible for the death of her daughter.

So how did I counsel her? At first I did not understand why the following words came out of my mouth until I reached the end of the story:

> "Upon my daughter's graduation from high school, I wrote an article that was published in the city newspaper about my experience as a mother letting go of her child. When my daughter was a toddler, I received a cryptic message from Above that my precious little girl was a gem. It was not until her high school graduation that I truly understood what that message meant.
>
> Our little children are not truly ours. They are little jewels on loan from Above for us to care for and nurture until it is time for them to leave home, like little birds from the nest. Then we must turn loose and return them to the Divine Creator, who takes them back to do with as deemed fit. Sometimes parents must turn loose of their little gems sooner than others and trust that the Divine Creator knows what is best."

With those words she seemed lighter and freer. Fortunately for this young woman, she released her sorrow and guilt early in life before they became deeply imbedded under layers of heavy foods and other pent-up emotions that accumulate throughout the years. When emotions that need to be released are stifled and suppressed deeply within, they can become toxic and adversely impact health and behavior, as the next case history demonstrates.

He was thirty-one years old with abdominal tumors. While his family wanted him to have the tumors surgically removed, he first wanted to try the program at the Institute.

He grew up with a mother who had agoraphobia (a fear of public places) and stated that life became hard when at one point in his childhood his mother had to work outside the home.

When he arrived, he appeared to be guarded and tense, suspicious of unknown smells or noises. While he had a handsome face and smooth skin, his jaw was firmly set, his eyes glinted, and he had a swollen abdomen.

One evening five days after his arrival, I led in a meditation class. As the students settled down on their yoga mats and drifted into relaxation, I softly and slowly told them it was safe to turn loose, relax, and let go. They slipped deeper into wonderful places – all but one person. The man with the abdominal tumors began to fidget and squirm. He rubbed his hands and then his feet. At length he sat up and waited for the meditation to end.

After class as students were leaving, he came to me to apologize for not being able to get into the meditation. He explained, however, that his hands started to itch uncomfortably, and then the itching moved to his feet. No amount of rubbing would stop it. Then the itching turned to burning, and he simply could not be still and slip into the meditation. I told him it was okay and that as his body relaxed during meditation, it may have been releasing burning toxins, perhaps from the abdomen.

So why did I say he may have been releasing poisons? When emotions, such as fear, control an individual's life, the body perceives a life-threatening situation, real or imagined. These emotions trigger adrenalin and other "fight or flight" hormones. Suddenly breathing becomes rapid and shallow to get more oxygen delivered throughout the body for speedy action. Blood goes from the digestive system to the brain for quick, alert thinking; to the heart for faster pumping; and to the muscles to fight or run. Meanwhile, as the digestive processes stop, the stomach knots up and holds undigested matter in the stomach (1).

This process continues until the individual perceives that the emergency has passed, and he or she is once again safe. Then the body shuts down the stress hormones, slips back into a relaxed mode, and breathes deeply and slowly. Blood reverts back to the gut, and digestion and other normal body processes that were put on hold continue as before (2).

Unfortunately, the hurried pace of life with its pressures and deadlines causes too many to feel that life is not safe enough to relax. They constantly remain "uptight" and ready for action. Food becomes hard to digest and stays trapped in the body indefinitely along with these emotions. A colonic hydrotherapist once told me that she saw shrimp come out of a man during a session. The man protested that he had not eaten shrimp in seven years!

From his mother the young man with the tumors inherited the feeling that the world is not a safe place. Through the years his stomach muscles may have been tightened and held in old trapped food matter and toxins along with fear, making digestion difficult. However, during the relaxation class he felt safe, relaxed, and let go of any anxiety and tensions, old food matter, and anything else which may have been trapped in his stomach for so long.

As the days wore on, his countenance began to soften, and so did his abdomen. At the end of the first week, he noticed his stomach felt soft instead of hard and knotted. At the end of the two-week program, his stomach was flat, his skin glowed, his eyes sparkled, and he was happy to return home to his family.

As this case history shows, emotions affect our health. When we are first born, we learn that milk removes hunger pangs and provides warmth and comfort. While growing up, eating patterns become ingrained from food cultures previously established in our families, such as grandma's good homemade cookies. And then social eating becomes a part of our lives as we use foods to celebrate happy events such as birthdays and Thanksgiving.

Have you ever watched a homely girl fall in love? Love is a powerfully healing force that opens up the body just as the warm sun brings out the blooms in flowers. Nutrient absorption becomes greatly enhanced. A bad complexion turns into a glowing rosy blush, the eyes sparkle, and the homely girl glows with loveliness (3).

On the other hand, foods can be detrimental, such as eating our favorite comfort foods to stuff unwanted feelings. For instance, each one of us has affection centers or areas in our brain where we experience love. If an individual is feeling a lack of love from the loss of a loved one, he or she may use a sweet treat such as candy to be lifted out of any sorrow and fill the void where the warm feelings from the loved one once dwelt. If he or she overwhelms the diet with sweets, then the excess sugar consumption can weaken the body and lower resistance to disease (4,5).

Also dark emotions can rob a body of nutrients. For example, rage can burn up sodium which is required for peristalsis. If it is not released, with time one may have digestive disturbances such as ulcers or irritable bowel syndrome (6).

A large proportion of the foods served at the Institute were greens and juices loaded with sodium and alkalizing minerals that fed the emotional as well as physical well-being of those following the program. We also instilled in the students that they were in a safe, loving place to promote healing.

Now for another case history.

She was thirty-eight years old and with her husband occupied Dr. Ann Wigmore's bedroom. Although they had completed the two-week program at a prior time, they had returned simply to rest and enjoy the lifestyle.

One of my directives was to check on and support the students and clientele, which I would do especially during the first week of the intensive cleansing program. It was at such a time while passing her on the veranda that I asked her how she was feeling.

She stated, "I feel all over as if I am dying. I can't shake it."

Stunned, I asked, "Have you mentioned this to your husband?"

"Yes, but he became alarmed and said, 'Don't say that!' But I can't help it. This feeling is all over me."

As she spoke, I mentally asked Above for the next words. The only answer that came to me was, "Have you experienced any trauma in the past?"

She stopped, reflected, and surprised me by saying, "Well, I had a miscarriage a year ago."

I responded, "You may be in the process of cleansing out old cell residue and debris lingering from the miscarriage."

Make no mistake about it - food and emotions are so intertwined as to be inseparable, and an individual cannot let go of one without letting go of the other. When one adopts a totally raw lifestyle, the foods are too lightweight to allow the "old stuff" to remain buried that has lurked in the recesses of the mind and driven thoughts and actions for years. In essence, one learns to forgive others, oneself, or life itself – simply by letting go.

It is here that the Laws of Nature change. No longer do the laws that govern the body on cooked foods apply to a body on totally raw and living foods. Instead, the mind and body transcend to a higher dimension of living where good health thrives and answers to life's questions become clear. It is here that one reconnects with oneself and the Divine Creator, and one heals not only emotionally and physically but spiritually as well.

Chapter 11
A Joyful Way of Life

It has been said that the spirit of the patient is far more important for healing than the work of any physician. The patient must choose deep within to live no matter how dire the disease (1). Dr. Ann Wigmore believed that as long as there is life in the patient, there is hope.

Certainly, western medicine has its place. I will be the first to say that it is necessary at times and has saved countless lives, including mine for which I will be forever grateful. But medicine can only help as far as the spirit and life force within the patient are strong enough to heal.

Neutraceuticals and nutritional food supplements can also be helpful when the body needs a boost, but their restorative powers are also limited to the spirit and life force within the patient.

However, the Living Foods Lifestyle® goes further. It not only restores the health of the patient but regenerates the life force and spirit within – be it human, animal, or plant.

Many feel so great after a week or two that they choose to stop all medications, but *never* do this without the supervision of a doctor. Others feel great after eliminating their life-threatening illness and think it is safe to return to their old habits. But be forewarned - this can be very dangerous. Lapsing into old patterns allows the return of the disease, and it does so with a strong vengeance.

While Wigmore was not the first to discover the beneficial powers of wheatgrass and enzymes, she was the first to promote indoor gardening and establish health retreats to teach a lifestyle necessary for healing and regeneration of the spirit.

My collection of case histories speaks for itself. I have researched and practiced many types of diets from the dregs of junk foods to the Standard American and Mediterranean diets to vegetarianism and veganism. Out of these I have seen none restore health and healing as does the Living Foods Lifestyle®. While many might argue that these cases are merely anecdotal and not sound scientific evidence, I find that science can be so slow that overwhelming anecdotal evidence precedes science. For this reason, I have chosen at least one case history from each category of health issues. Certainly, raw veganism and the Living Foods Lifestyle® beg for research not only for mankind but the whole Earth as well.

Stop and think - if this lifestyle is so powerful that it can bring an unresponsive dying dog lying limply at death's door to greet the guardian with jumping joy the very next morning, then how powerfully healing this lifestyle must be for the whole Earth. At the Institute I was amazed at how very little packaging is required to feed so many. Also the natural wastes created from such a lifestyle are renewable and go back into Mother Earth for future generations and healings.

As Leola once told me, "Instead of seeing the glass half empty, suddenly it seems three-quarters full" (2). When is the last time you felt like skipping and jumping for the sheer joy of it?

The Living Foods Lifestyle® is not just a fad – it is a path to healing not only for mankind but for the whole Earth as well. It is not easy to do it one hundred percent. It requires much work, discipline, and perseverance to sacrifice cooked, dead pseudofoods and liquids that one *thinks* he or she needs "to keep going."

But I must warn you – should you adopt this lifestyle one hundred percent, you will never be the same again. It is like driving a Rolls Royce; you never want to go back to a Ford or Chevrolet again.

Chapter 12
Cleansing and Healing Menus

All raw foods are cleansing and healing, but some are more so than others. In a life-threatening illness it is very important to choose and prepare raw and living foods in a way that expedites the healing process. Juiced and blended foods tend to work best.

Stop and think - solid matter, such as improperly chewed food, has its own definite shape. When dumped into the stomach, the elastic gastrointestinal tract has to become distorted, convoluted, and bent out of shape to accommodate such foods. Years of eating solid, improperly chewed, cooked foods drain the energy and life out of the digestive tract until peristalsis becomes sluggish and increasingly slows down. The passage of food takes longer and becomes lodged and trapped, creating fermentation and bloating as well as a great habitat for harmful bacteria, parasites, and microorganisms to breed infection and disease.

On the other hand, a liquid takes on the shape of its container. Thus, a light diet of juices and blended foods takes on the shape of the digestive tract. It does not get distorted and bent out of shape just to push matter through the system. Instead, it can relax and rest.

Blended foods are already mechanically broken down and predigested with good bacteria when rejuvelac is added, so the gut can rest during the process. Raw juices are great for soaking up and sloughing off encrusted matter beyond the reach of colon flushes. Plus a relaxed gastrointestinal tract turns loose and lets go of old matter that needs to be released. What a boost this is for a diseased digestive tract that is too weak to properly function.

The following are healing menus for seven days. The menus for the first three days offer juiced and blended foods that allow time for the body to turn around and orient itself from poor health to healing. After the three-day detoxifying period, the body becomes ready for crunchy solid food, but it needs to be done carefully. Immediately going into heavy solids can be stressful for the gut and create uncomfortable detoxification symptoms. Thus, the menu for day four is designed to gradually lead the body out of liquid foods into whole foods. The menu for days 5, 6, and 7 provides for raw gourmet foods which can be consumed on a daily basis using various raw recipes.

Starting the second week of the program and thereafter, juiced and blended foods one day a week followed by six days of whole raw foods will continue the cleansing and healing process. While it takes time, one will be rewarded by the positive changes felt and seen in the body.

NOTE: Too much time is spent counting portions, serving sizes, calories, carbohydrates, protein, and fats when the focus should be on foods dense with alkalizing minerals, enzymes, antioxidants, and other live phytochemicals vital for healing. Living foods includes these phytochemicals and others both known and unknown to science and have a dramatically greater nutritional profile than their conventional counterparts. Therefore, one does not have to eat as many calories with living foods to get the body's required nutrition. But do feel free to eat as much as you wish without the guilt of conventional foods.

The recipes for the menus are listed in chapter 13 with explanations of the importance of each and their healing properties. And be certain to consume lots of fresh purified water, rejuvelac (when appropriate), and raw juices every day to flush toxins from the body and enhance the process.

Day 1

Upon Arising
2 oz. fresh squeezed wheat grass juice
OR warm water or rejuvelac with fresh-squeezed lemon
- followed by breakfast 1/2 hour later

Breakfast
Fresh-squeezed juice of carrots, beets, celery, and leafy greens
OR Energy Soup

Lunch
Buckwheat Porridge

Supper
Green Pudding
OR Fruit Smoothie

Snacks
Purified water or rejuvelac

Day 2

Upon Arising
2 oz. fresh squeezed wheat grass juice
OR warm water or rejuvelac with fresh-squeezed lemon
- followed by breakfast 1/2 hour later

Breakfast
Fresh-squeezed juice of carrots, beets, celery, and leafy greens
OR Energy Soup

Lunch
Sesame Shake

Supper
Green Pudding

Snacks
Purified water or rejuvelac

Day 3
<u>Upon Arising</u>
Fresh squeezed wheat grass juice
OR warm water or rejuvelac with fresh-squeezed lemon
- followed by breakfast 1/2 hour later

<u>Breakfast</u>
Fresh-squeezed juice of carrots, beets, celery, and leafy greens
OR Energy Soup

<u>Lunch</u>
Buckwheat Porridge

<u>Supper</u>
Fruit Smoothie
OR Sesame Shake

<u>Snacks</u>
Purified water or rejuvelac

Day 4
<u>Upon Arising</u>
2 oz. fresh squeezed wheat grass juice
OR warm water or rejuvelac with fresh-squeezed lemon
- followed by breakfast 1/2 hour later

<u>Breakfast</u>
Fresh-squeezed juice of carrots, beets, celery, and leafy greens
OR Energy Soup

<u>Lunch</u>
Onion Kraut with Avocado

<u>Supper</u>
Fruit Smoothie
OR Green Pudding

<u>Snacks</u>
Bananas, apples, pineapple, or any favorite Fruit

Days 5, 6, & 7

Upon Arising
2 oz. fresh squeezed wheat grass juice
OR warm water or rejuvelac with fresh-squeezed lemon
- followed by breakfast 1/2 hour later

Breakfast
Fresh-squeezed juice of carrots, beets, celery, and leafy greens

Lunch
Squash Spaghetti with vegetables
        and Pesto or Marinara sauce*
        OR
Stuffed bell pepper* with any of the following:
        - guacamole
        - Cheesy White Sauce
        OR
Shepherd's pie*
        OR
Salad with Avocado dressing*
        OR
Pizza*
        OR
Onion Kraut with Avocado
        OR
Vegetable Pattie*

Supper
Fruit Smoothie
OR Green Pudding
OR Energy Soup

Snacks
Crackers, cookies, or favorite fruits

* Any of these entrees can be followed by a dish of chopped pineapple.
The enzymes in pineapple aid in the digestion of lunch meals.

Chapter 13 -
Cleansing and Healing Recipes

The following are recipes for the above menus plus desserts to carry one through holidays, potlucks, and other get-togethers where cooked food is served. These recipes are designed simply as a guide for creating your favorite raw dishes and may be altered to suit your needs and tastes.

I have included pink Himalayan salt in a few of the recipes. Himalayan salt is unrefined with many essential minerals intact which are required by the body.

Many physicians call salt (sodium chloride) a poison to the body, especially the white refined kind. However, once the sodium is cleaved from the chloride in the salt, the chloride may combine with the hydrogen molecule in the body to form hydrochloric acid in the stomach. Hydrochloric acid breaks down protein and kills harmful organisms that may be on foods. Many people, especially when they get older, tend to have a hydrochloric acid deficiency. Therefore, a few granules under the tongue several days apart may aid digestion.

However, some people have salt sensitivities from the best salts, and even nama shoyu and dulse may create reactions. For these people I strongly urge omitting salt, nama shoyu, or dulse unless otherwise instructed by your physician.

Do keep in mind that the rules for preparing raw foods are different than for cooked. Cooking destroys the original flavors in foods. To make cooked foods palatable, salt, spices, and condiments are added.

On the other hand, raw foods retain their inherent flavors, requiring little, if any, salt, spices, or condiments. And unlike cooked foods, the final flavors in raw dishes may need adjusting as the flavor varies depending upon the soil where the ingredients are grown.

Be open-minded. One may be pleasantly surprised to find that foods that taste unappealing when cooked are very delightful in the raw state. And do not be surprised if you find that your body starts demanding foods that your taste buds never allowed. A journey on a totally raw foods diet brings many delightful surprises.

Enjoy!

Namaste.

Rejuvelac
(from the kitchens of the Ann Wigmore Foundation® and Ann Wigmore Natural Health Institute)

This delightful drink is concentrated with predigested nutrition, enzymes, antioxidants, probiotics, and other nutrients, making nutritional absorption much easier. When used as a base in soups, smoothies, and puddings in lieu of water, the concentration of antioxidants gives soups and smoothies a longer shelf life.

Ingredients:
2 cups quinoa or other grain

Pour grain in a 1-gallon jar and cover with 4 cups clean filtered water. Cover mouth of jar with mesh held in place with a rubber band and let stand 5 or more hours. Then pour off water and rinse. Let drain by standing jar at a tilt in a drain rack. As grain falls down the side of jar, make certain there is enough space for air to reach inside to keep grain from souring. Rinse 2 or 3 times a day and let stand at a tilt until little tails grow. (Sometimes the tails in quinoa do not fully grow until they have soaked in the first batch of rejuvelac.)

After the tails appear, rinse the grains a few times to wash out any bad bacteria. Then fill the gallon jar through the mesh up to its neck with clean filtered water and let stand one to two days. When the water is cloudy and the top bubbly, the first batch of rejuvelac is ready for harvest. Pour off the liquid into a container and refrigerate.
Yield: 1/2 to 3/4 gallon.

Next fill the jar through the mesh up to its neck with pure filtered water for a second batch of rejuvelac. After a day or two, simply pour into another container and refrigerate. The grains will support 2 to 3 healthy batches of rejuvelac that will last a week or two in the refrigerator, depending upon the weather. The seeds can be thrown into a compost heap or a flower bed. Birds tend to ignore the spent seeds since most of the nutrition and life has been leeched out.

Variations: Try adding fresh-squeezed ginger and lemon juice or squeezing strawberries into rejuvulac for different flavors.

NOTE: For no apparent reason, a batch may sometime turn rotten or foul smelling. Instead of discarding it, water flowers and plants with it. In a couple of weeks plants will be covered with blooms and leaves. Plants are also starved for good nutrition.

CAUTION: When drunk on an empty stomach, rejuvelac can raise blood sugar levels in type 1 diabetics but without noticeable affect in type 2's. On the other hand, both types 1 and 2 diabetics tolerate rejuvelac very well in soups and smoothies. Also in cases of candida, rejuvelac may increase symptoms at first until the body is cleansed and the yeast is in check.

Raw Fresh-Squeezed Juice
(from the kitchen of Linda Ruff)

Next to wheatgrass juice, raw vegetable and fruit juices are probably the most powerfully energizing, cleansing, and healing of foods. Raw juices supply the body with concentrated nutrition, enzymes, antioxidants, and other phytochemicals, and when leafy greens are added, they help stabilize blood sugar levels during a fast. They soak up and escort old matter out of the gut while stimulating peristalsis in a weakened digestive tract. They also clean higher in the body where colon hydrotherapy cannot reach. Raw juices on a daily basis hydrate and "youth" the face, skin, and body.

The following ingredients make a very powerful drink. Carrots are highly concentrated with the antioxidant beta-carotene which is great for clearing blurry eyesight and creating sharper vision. Beets and beet greens break down acid material such as stones in the urinary bladder, liver, and gallbladder. Celery replenishes electrolytes and is an excellent source of sodium required for peristalsis. Greens alkalize the body while building up the blood, and aloe vera soothes a distressed digestive tract.

For best results, juices should be consumed daily on an empty stomach, such as first thing in the morning 1/2 hour before eating or as a breakfast.

Ingredients:
1 pound raw carrots
1/4 beet
1 stalk celery with leaves

1-2 bunches of a combination of greens such as spinach, chard, kale, dandelion, plantain, clover, sunflower, or other greens
3" large or 4-6" thin aloe vera leaf

Rinse and clean produce. Run through a juicer. If using a centrifugal juicer, let it run for several minutes afterward to extract most of the juice. The pulp should be dry.
Yield: 1½ to 2 cups.

Variation: Try juicing apple and cucumber with greens for a unique flavor.

Buckwheat Porridge
(from the kitchen of Linda Ruff)

Buckwheat is gluten free and supplies all of the essential amino acids, making it a good meat substitute. It is a good source of the bioflavonoid rutin, which strengthens capillaries and blood vessels, and is necessary for vitamin C to function. Dates have been used for chest and throat sickness, and its fiber makes it a far healthier sweetener than refined sugars. Cinnamon is a warming spice that aids in blood sugar stabilization. Banana gives the cereal a smooth, creamy texture, and the blueberries are loaded with antioxidants and strengthen vision. The flax or hemp oil adds the omega-3 fatty acid and keeps the buckwheat cereal from being drying to the body.

Ingredients:
1/2 cup buckwheat groats soaked
 in filtered water a few hours
2 pitted dates, soaked in filtered
 water overnight
OR 1/2 teaspoon raw honey
1-2 tablespoons flax or hemp oil
1/2 teaspoon cinnamon
1 banana
Blueberries to taste

Drain the soak water from the buckwheat groats and rinse. Blend with the raw honey or dates and soak water, flax or hemp oil, cinnamon, and banana until smooth. It may be necessary to add water for a pureed consistency. Add some blueberries and pulse.

Yield: Approximately 1 1/2 cups.

Variations: Other grains and seeds with complete protein, such as millet, quinoa, or sunflower, can be substituted for buckwheat. Also other fruits, such as apples or strawberries, can be used.

NOTE: Over a period of time buckwheat can be drying and bleach out the skin. Cows fed buckwheat have been found to sunburn easily.

Energy Soup
(from the kitchens of the Ann Wigmore Foundation® and the Ann Wigmore Natural Health Institute)

Along with wheatgrass juice and rejuvelac, this soup was a very significant part of the healing program at the Institute. It was readily available for students and staff in the dining room at all hours day or night.

With rejuvelac, Energy Soup is easily digested and provides all of the nutritional needs for the body in one dish. The sunflower and buckwheat greens used in the soup were raised in the greenhouse to provide lots of chlorophyll, alkalizing minerals, vitamins, and light weight protein. The sprouts contain exponential amounts of nutrition, fiber, and predigested carbohydrates and protein. Dulse or kelp provide minerals. The avocado provides good fats necessary for the body to utilize vitamins A, D, E, and K without cholesterol and gives the soup a creamy texture. The sweet potato or squash add the antioxidant beta-carotene. Non-genetically modified papaya is rich in enzymes, vitamins and minerals and great for aiding digestion, which is a very important part of the healing process.

Ingredients:
12 oz. rejuvelac or filtered water
1 teaspoon dulse or kelp
1 avocado
Some chunks of yellow squash or sweet potato
1 apple
OR some chunks of papaya
Sunflower and/or buckwheat greens
Mixed sprouts (e.g., alfalfa, red clover, fenugroek, broccoli, onion)

Blend the first five ingredients. Then add the sprouts and greens to make a creamy pudding. Eat half in a bowl and store the other half in the refrigerator to be eaten the next day.

Yield: approximately 4 cups.

NOTE: The antioxidants in rejuvelac retard spoilage and will extend shelf life longer than 24 hours. If water is used instead of rejuvelac, the soup should be eaten immediately as it will oxidize rapidly.

NOTE: At the Institute, Energy Soup was not kept more than 24 hours. If any was left over from the previous day, it was dehydrated into crackers called "crummies." These were great added to Energy Soup or given to the students to eat on their travels home.

NOTE: Many with parasites, cancer, or yeast infections cannot tolerate any sweet fruits. For this reason, eliminate the papaya and use only green apple until these conditions are eliminated or in proper balance.

NOTE: Since many with cancer or yeast infections preferred not to eat sweet fruits in their Energy Soup, papaya was served on the side at the Institute. Also seed cheeses and yogurt were served on the side which made excellent flavor enhancers.

Seed Cheese
(from the kitchens of the Ann Wigmore Foundation® and the Ann Wigmore Natural Health Institute)

The following cheese and yogurt recipes are delicious and a good substitute for dairy. They are cultured for easy digestion and a good source of probiotics and antioxidants. The calcium is more easily digested than the calcium in dairy.

Ingredients:
1 cup Rejuvelac or filtered water
2 cups hulled raw sunflower, pumpkin,
   or sesame seeds

Soak seeds for 8 hours and sprout up to 8 hours. (Sesame seeds should be soaked about 3 hours.) After this time, pour Rejuvelac into a blender. If rejuvelac is not available, use filtered water. Blend at high speed, slowly adding seeds until all are blended to a smooth paste (approximately 4 minutes). Pour the mixture into a glass jar, cover with a cloth or towel, and set aside for 3-8 hours.* If using a sprout bag, pour the mixture into the bag and hang over a bowl for 3 to 6 hours.* (If using water, then let ferment 2 extra hours.) After the time frame has elapsed, pour off the whey from the jar. The cheese should be stored tightly covered in the refrigerator and should last 5 days.
Yield: Approximately 2½ cups.

*Length of time depends upon the climate. NOTE: One can use ¼ cup from a previous batch to mix with the new batch.

Seed Yogurt
(From the kitchens of the Ann Wigmore Foundation® and the Ann Wigmore Natural Health Institute)
Ingredients:
2 cups Rejuvelac or filtered water
2 cups hulled raw sunflower,
   pumpkin, or sesame seeds
Follow the same procedure as for Seed Cheese using a jar. Set aside for 3 to 6 hours, depending upon the climate, and retain the liquid. Stir and refrigerate.
Yield: Approximately 4 cups.

Green Soup
(adapted from the Energy Soup recipe at the Ann Wigmore
Foundation® and the Ann Wigmore Natural Health Institute)

This soup is a powerful cleanser and healer of any illness in the body. It is dense in most nutrients that humankind requires, making it a meal all in one. It takes on the shape of the digestive tract and promotes peristalsis and healing.

The concentration of enzymes and probiotics in the rejuvelac predigests the ingredients, making the nutrients easily absorbed by the body. Dulse or kelp provides minerals, and avocado makes a creamy soup while providing an excellent source of fats and protein. The papaya and squash provide the antioxidant beta-carotene, and the greens balance the sugars in the fruit and promote healthy blood. The mixture of sprouts provides an excellent variety of exponential nutrition, the apple provides pectin, which aids digestion and neutralizes toxins in the body, and cinnamon helps to stabilize blood sugar levels, alleviate stress, and warm the body in the winter.

Ingredients:
12 oz. rejuvelac or filtered water
1 teaspoon dulse or kelp
1 teaspoon cinnamon
1 avocado
Some chunks of yellow squash
1 apple
Some chunks of papaya
Combination of greens such as lettuce, spinach, chard, kale, dandelion, plantain, clover, sunflower, or other greens
Mixed sprouts (e.g., alfalfa, red clover, fenugroek, broccoli, onion)

Blend all ingredients until thick like a pudding and smooth. Eat half in a bowl and store the other half in the refrigerator to be eaten the next day.
Yield: approximately 4 cups.

NOTE: The antioxidants in rejuvelac retard spoilage and will extend shelf life up to 24 hours. If water is used instead of rejuvelac, the soup should be eaten immediately as it will oxidize rapidly.

VARIATION: Instead of cinnamon try substituting 1/2 tsp. each basil and oregano and add a clove of garlic. Or try mixing in some Raw Applesauce or Cheesy White Sauce (the recipes follow) to complement the soup.

NOTE: For a yeast infection or cancer, eliminate the papaya and use only green apple.

Sesame Shake
(adapted from a recipe at the Ann Wigmore Foundation® and the Ann Wigmore Natural Health Institute)

This shake is *so* satisfying and nourishing. The sesame seeds are an excellent source of calcium and used far better by the body than calcium from dairy. This shake provided excellent results as part of a healing program prescribed by a doctor for a patient with diverticulitis, who was deficient in calcium.

Ingredients:
1/2 cup sesame seeds
2 dates
3-4 bananas
1/4-1/2 teaspoon cinnamon

Soak 2 dates in filtered water overnight. Soak ½ cup sesame seeds in filtered water for 3 hours. Pour off soak water from the sesame seeds and blend with the dates and soak water, cinnamon, and 3-4 bananas (depending upon desired thickness). It may be necessary to add some water for blending.
Yield: approximately 4 cups.

Green Pudding
(from the kitchen of Linda Ruff)

This pudding is always a hit at my workshops and great for those who do not like to eat vegetables. The mango improves digestion and kidney function and helps clear up the skin. The banana feeds the nerves and good bacteria in the gut, and avocado provides healthy fats and protein. The greens stabilize sugar levels and oxygenate the blood. The sprouts boost the nutrient profile of this delicious food, and rejuvelac provides for easy digestion.

Ingredients:
1 mango
1 banana
1 avocado
Combination of greens (kale, spinach, dandelion, etc.)
Mixed sprouts (e.g., alfalfa, red clover, fenugroek, broccoli, onion)
Enough rejuvelac or water to cover blades in blender

Blend all ingredients until the consistency of a thick pudding. Enjoy!
Yield: 2-3 cups.

NOTE: If water is used as a base, the green smoothie needs to be consumed immediately as the air oxidizes it rapidly. If, however, rejuvelac is used, the high levels of antioxidants give it a longer shelf life, and a batch will last up to twenty-four hours or more.

NOTE: Mango may be substituted for your favorite fruit.

Fruit Smoothie
(from the kitchen of Linda Ruff)

While greens and vegetables support growth, repair, and maintenance of the body, fruits promote cleansing. After a day of greens, the body sometimes needs something from the opposite end of the spectrum to balance digestion and promote peristalsis, and fruits fill this need. A fruit smoothie at the end of the day prepares the body for its nightly cleansing processes.

Just like watermelon, a cooling fruit smoothie provides a great boost when feeling tired and drained. Fruits are high in antioxidants and potassium, another mineral required for peristalsis. Bananas add thickness and give a rich creamy texture. With rejuvelac a fruit smoothie soaks up and pulls sludge out of the body. With time the stomach will flatten out.

Ingredients:
8 oz. rejuvelac, coconut water,
   or raw apple juice
Fresh frozen fruits or berries
1-2 bananas

Blend all ingredients into a thick consistency.
Yield: approximately 3 cups.

Onion Kraut with Avocado
(from the kitchen of Julie Jewel)

Clients with irritable bowel and other digestive disorders find this recipe very soothing to their digestive tract. Also it is a wonderful food with which to break a fast.

When pink Himalayan salt is added, raw kraut provides the three things required for digestion: 1) enzymes, 2) probiotics, and 3) material to manufacture stomach acid for digesting protein. Kraut is fermented at room temperature which is Mother Nature's way of cooking and predigesting for easy absorption. The cabbage used to make kraut should be prepared within hours of harvest while it still glistens with life and is heavy with its natural water content. This water is necessary for fermentation. Without it, it will turn brown and be dry. If the head has not been recently harvested, water may need to be added. The onion helps to sweeten the kraut as well as lend flavor. The dulse or kelp and Himalayan salt provide minerals, and avocado makes the kraut taste smooth, rich, and creamy as well as provide good fats and protein.

Ingredients:
1 large or 2 smaller heads of fresh cabbage
1 large onion
1-2 cups water (optional)
1/2 chopped avocado
Dulse or kelp
Pink Himalayan salt to taste, if tolerated

Remove and save three or four outer leaves of cabbage. Shred, grate, or food process the remaining cabbage and onion into tiny pieces and put into a crock or large bowl. With a mallet pound the cabbage until the juices are squeezed out. For older cabbage water may need to be added. Cover with the saved outer leaves of cabbage. Place a plate with a heavy weight on top to squeeze the juices out of the cabbage as it ferments. Set aside for 2 to 4 days, depending on the weather. It is ready when the cabbage has cultured down and the juice comes to the top. In warm weather a rank smell may emanate from the kraut, indicating it is getting ready for harvest. Harvest by removing the weight and outer leaves. The top surface of the harvested kraut may be darker but is edible according to Wigmore. The juice can be drunk or kept with the kraut stored in a glass bowl with lid.

When ready to eat, put in a bowl and add the chopped avocado. Sprinkle with dulse or kelp and Himalayan salt (if tolerated) and serve. *Yield:* approximately 5-6 cups.

NOTE: Omit the salt and dulse if they affect blood pressure or create other health issues.

Veggie Patty
(from the kitchen of Linda Ruff)

Many ask what to do with the dried pulp left from juicing. Simply toss it into a compost pile or flower garden or use the pulp to make burgers and meatless balls. A burger is very filling, and the pulp is an excellent source of vegetables for those who will not eat them.

Sunflower seeds are rich in vitamins, including the sunshine vitamin D, and provide fats and all of the essential amino acids for protein found in meat. The onion has antiobiotic properties that fight infections and helps rid the body of heavy metals and parasites. Dulse provides minerals, and curry powder increases metabolism and restores good breathing.

Ingredients:
2 cups carrot pulp from juicing
2 cups ground sunflower seeds
1 large onion, finely chopped
2 tablespoons nama shoyu*, if tolerated
OR Himalayan salt, if tolerated
1 teaspoon dulse powder
1 teaspoon curry powder

Combine ingredients in a bowl and mix well. Form into patties or balls.
Yield: 10-12 patties.

NOTE: When dehydrated, they turn brown to look just like cooked burgers, but keep in mind - dried foods pull much moisture from the body.

* Nama shoyu means unpasteurized soy sauce in Japanese and may be very high in salt and MSG. For those with salt sensitivities omit nama shoyu.

Squash Spaghetti
(from the kitchen of Linda Ruff)

Spaghetti made from zucchini, summer, or butternut squash makes a great substitute for those with gluten intolerance and wheat sensitivities. It has a sweet flavor and provides the antioxidants beta-carotene and vitamin A, which fight infection and support vision. Squash alkalizes the blood and liver. It supplies many nutrients and is easy to digest. Squash and pumpkin seeds expel roundworms and tapeworms.

Ingredients:
Zucchini, summer, or butternut squash
Olive oil
Parsley flakes

Run squash through a spaghetti maker or a vegetable spiralizer. Then coat with olive oil and garnish with parsley flakes on top.
Yield: 1 large or 2 small zucchini squashes serves 2-3.

VARIATIONS: Add vegetables such as chopped red and orange bell pepper, broccoli, green beans, sliced onion, sliced mushrooms marinaded in nama shoyu*, and other vegetables and stir in a marinara, pesto, or white sauce made with nuts.

* Nama shoyu is Japanese for soy sauce.

NOTE: Vegetable spiralizers may be purchased online.

Pesto Sauce
(from the kitchen of Linda Ruff)

Pesto sauce has ingredients that supply many beneficial properties for the body. Basil is good for stabilizing blood sugar levels, stomach disturbances, and constipation. Olive oil helps to dissolve stones and break down hardened matter, making it a mild and effective laxative. Garlic aids digestion and the lymph system in eliminating toxic metals, worms, and parasites. The pine nuts replace parmesan cheese and are an excellent source of protein for replacing meat. Spinach and greens provide cleansing chlorophyll along with the basil and add more bulk to the sauce.

Ingredients:
1/4 cup olive oil
3 large or 4 small cloves garlic
1/2 cup pine nuts
1 bunch fresh basil
1 bunch spinach or other leafy green

Blend thoroughly.
Yield: 4-5 servings.

NOTE: This makes a great pizza sauce for those with arthritis and sensitivities to tomatoes and other nightshade plants.

VARIATION: ¼ cup nutritional yeast flakes may be substituted for the pine nuts for a cheesy flavor.

Pizza

Clients think they will never get to eat pasta, spaghetti, or pizza again on a raw vegan diet but are pleasantly surprised to find they do not have to forego these foods. The following recipes offer raw versions that will please everyone's taste buds, including those of omnivores.

Buckwheat Crust
(from the kitchen of Linda Ruff)

Buckwheat is a good protein substitute for meat and gluten-free for those with gluten intolerance and wheat sensitivities. It is also a good source of the bioflavonoid rutin, which strengthens capillaries and blood vessels and is necessary for vitamin C to function. Flaxseed provides an excellent source of omega-3 fatty acid and is another complete protein with all of the essential amino acids. It helps to hold the buckwheat crust together and keep it from crumbling. The olive oil provides moisture and also helps hold the crust together. Basil has antibacterial and antifungal properties that fight infections and parasites. Oregano is good for digestion and helps eliminate poisons from the body.

Ingredients:
1 1/4 cups raw hulled buckwheat groats,
  soaked 6 hours to make 2 1/2 cups
1/3 cup extra-virgin cold-pressed olive oil
3 tablespoons ground flaxseeds
3 tablespoons nama shoyu, if tolerated
1 tablespoon dried basil
1 tablespoon dried oregano

Blend the soaked buckwheat, nama shoyu, olive oil, basil, and oregano and pour into a bowl. Stir in the ground flaxseeds to thicken until a dough is formed. With a large spoon, shape the dough onto a dehydrator sheet and put on a dehydrator tray. Form four 6- or 7-inch rounds that are approximately 1/4-inch thick. Dehydrate overnight and turn them the next morning to finish drying.
Yield: 4 6- or 7-inch pizza crusts.

VARIATIONS: Can be shaped into crackers as well. Simply spread dough into desired shape, sprinkle with Himalayan salt (if tolerated), and cut into desired shape.

Marinara Sauce
(from the kitchen of Linda Ruff)

Tomatoes act as an antiseptic and are alkalizing for the body. Roma tomatoes pack less water and make a thicker sauce. When eaten raw, tomatoes reduce hepatitis and cirrhosis of the liver. They provide vitamin A and lycopene, a powerful antioxidant. Fresh garlic fights influenza and amoebic dysentery. Oregano fights viruses. On top of its beneficial properties, fresh basil relieves itching from insect bites and skin eruptions when applied directly to the skin. Bell peppers provide more vitamin C than oranges. Mushrooms offer vitamins and minerals and lack sugar, making it a good choice for diabetics.

Ingredients:
3 cups fresh Roma tomatoes
4-5 cloves garlic, minced
Dried basil to taste
Dried oregano to taste
1 1/2 cups dehydrated tomatoes
OR 4 tablespoons ground flaxseeds
1 tablespoon Nama shoyu, if tolerated

Blend all ingredients and allow mixture to sit for approximately 10 minutes to soften the dehydrated tomatoes or allow the ground flaxseeds to thicken.
Yield: approximately 3 1/2 cups.

VARIATION: The pizza crust tastes excellent covered with vegetables and topped with pesto sauce!

Vegetable Toppings:
Chopped fresh greens of basil, arugula, spinach, and others
Thinly sliced onion rings
Chopped red, yellow, and green bell pepper
Sliced olives
Sliced mushrooms, marinated in nama shoyu for half an hour,
  if tolerated
Seed Cheese
OR Cheesy White Sauce

To assemble the pizza: Place the tomato topping on each crust. Top with the fresh greens, onion rings, mushrooms, olives, and bell pepper. Crumble on top bits of Seed Cheese or Cheesy White Sauce that has set up in the refrigerator.
Yield: 4 6- or 7-inch pizzas.

NOTE: Bell peppers and tomatoes are members of the nightshade family and may aggravate arthritis symptoms. Pesto sauce is an excellent substitute for marinara sauce.

Cheesy White Sauce
(from the kitchen of Linda Ruff)

This versatile recipe can be used as a creamy white sauce or as a fermented cheese full of good bacteria.

Ingredients:
1 1/2 cups unpasteurized almonds
OR macadamias
2 tablespoons extra-virgin cold-pressed olive oil
3 tablespoons nutritional yeast flakes
Fresh-squeezed juice of 1/2 lemon
Himalayan salt to taste, if tolerated
1/2 cup rejuvelac
OR water, as necessary

Soak the almonds or macadamias in 2 1/2 cups of filtered water overnight. The almonds should have the brown skins removed. Combine with the remaining ingredients and add enough rejuvelac or water to blend into a cheesy sauce. Set in the refrigerator for 24 hours to thicken. Remove and drop small amounts over pizza.
Yield: 1 1/2 cups.

VARIATIONS: For a living fermented cheese, place mixture in a mesh bag and hang over a bowl or line a sieve with cheesecloth and cover. Allow to rest for approximately 24 hours or until the whey or liquid has dripped out, and the mixture has firmed. The Seed Cheese recipe above can also be used.

NOTE: There are two methods of pasteurization: 1) heat-treated at high temperatures and 2) injected with a chemical. Unpasteurized almonds may need to be shipped direct from the grower.

NOTE: For a creamy sauce over burgers, meatless balls, spaghetti, and other creations, add more rejuvelac or water and blend to desired consistency.

NOTE: For a flavorful sauce or cheese, add 4-5 cloves of medium-sized garlic and 1/3 cup lemon juice, or simply add your favorite herbs and spices and stuff bell peppers or mushrooms with the sauce or cheese.

Marinaded Vegetable Dish
(from the kitchen of Linda Ruff)

In the summertime I love to frequent the farmer's markets and local growers for live organic vegetables and combine them in a dish with a marinade of olive oil and herbs. The combination of vegetables in this dish provides a large biodiversity of beneficial antioxidants and phytochemicals. The high fiber content feeds the good bacteria and scrubs out the digestive system which flattens the stomach.

Ingredients:
1 cup extra-virgin cold-pressed olive oil
1/4 cup raw cider vinegar
1/4 cup raw honey
2 teaspoons each of sage,
    rosemary, and thyme
OR rosemary with crushed garlic
OR sage with crushed onion
OR oregano and basil
Zucchini, summer, or butternut squash,
    sliced or spiralized into spaghetti
Green beans
Mushrooms
Chopped eggplant
Red and orange bell peppers
Tomatoes
Sliced onion rings
Other available vegetables
1 tablespoon dulse flakes

Blend olive oil, raw cider vinegar, raw honey, and your choice of herbs into a marinade. Wash and chop the vegetables to desired size and combine in a bowl.   Pour the marinade and sprinkle dulse over the vegetables until well coated. Let sit for a few hours or overnight until ready to serve.
Yield: 4-5 cups.

NOTE: Eggplant, bell peppers, and tomatoes are members of the nightshade family and may irritate arthritis symptoms.

Raw Vegetable Soup
(from the kitchen of Linda Ruff)

This soup tastes great and reminds me of the cooked version I love in the winter. It can be heated *only* until warm to the touch for chilly days. Simply place a bowl of soup in a pan of hot water for 5-15 minutes and stir occasionally until it warms up.

Ingredients:
4 or 5 fresh tomatoes
1/2 large onion
5 cloves peeled garlic
1 tablespoon dried basil
1 tablespoon dried oregano
1/2 peeled lemon
2 tablespoons olive oil
Combination of green beans,
   sliced or spiralized squash,
   corn cut from three cobs,
   fresh shelled peas, broccoli,
   chopped red and yellow bell peppers,
   and other freshly harvested
   vegetables
Dulse or pink Himalayan salt to taste, if tolerated

Combine the first seven ingredients in a blender or Vita-Mix and blend until smooth. Pour in a bowl and add the assorted vegetables. Add dulse to taste, if tolerated.

NOTE: Eggplant, bell peppers, and tomatoes are members of the nightshade family and may irritate arthritis symptoms.

Raw Shepherd's Pie
(from the kitchen of Linda Ruff)

This is a satisfying dish full of a variety of nutrients, especially when fresh produce is in season at farmer's markets and local growers. It keeps for several days in the refrigerator and packs well for lunches on the go.

Ingredients:
Sliced fresh vegetables in season
  (squash, tomatoes, green onions,
  peas, corn, green beans, okra,
  broccoli, cauliflower, bell
  peppers, etc.)
Sliced mushrooms marinaded in
  nama shoyu, if tolerated
1 cup Cheesy White Sauce
WITH sage and onion
OR lemon and garlic
OR oregano and basil
OR sage, rosemary, and thyme
OR your favorite herbs and spices
Dulse flakes

Chop or slice vegetables to desired size and place in a casserole dish. Add the sliced mushrooms. Add your favorite herbs and spices to the cheesy white sauce to make a thick cover over the vegetables. Sprinkle dulse flakes on top.
Yield: 5-6 servings.

Avocado Dressing
(from the kitchen of Linda Ruff)

A student in my home came up with this recipe, and I love it to this day. Avocados have a compatible pH with the body, are an excellent source of easily digested organic fats and protein, and improve hair and skin when consumed regularly. Leeks are an excellent source of the carotenoids lutein and zeaxanthin, both of which are good for vision, and their flavor is milder than onions, which makes it less hazardous to your social life.

Ingredients:
2 avocados
1 inch piece of leek

Add enough rejuvelac or water to cover blades and blend until thick and fluffy. The fats in avocado oxidize rapidly, so the dressing should be eaten immediately.
Yield: approximately 1 1/2 cups.

Raw Miso Dressing
(from the kitchen of Linda Ruff)

This dressing is good when fresh produce is not available and makes an excellent marinade. Miso is a fermented product with nutrients of enzymes and microorganisms that promote good digestion; vitamins and minerals, including B_{12}; and properties that block radioactive absorption. However, the miso must be unpasteurized for the body to benefit from these properties. Raw cider vinegar is high in potassium and prevents joint stiffness. Raw unpasteurized honey contains enzymes and fights allergies and inflammation.

Ingredients:
2 tablespoons unpasteurized organic miso
2 tablespoons raw cider vinegar
1 tablespoon raw honey
3 tablespoons filtered water

Blend all ingredients and serve.

Yield: About 1/3 cup.

Raw Raspberry Vinaigrette
(from the kitchen of Linda Ruff)

This dressing is good on salads and as a marinade. The high potassium level in the raw cider vinegar promotes peristalsis which aids digestion and dissolves acid crystals which are deposited in the joints, creating bursitis, arthritis, and rheumatism. The malic acid in the vinegar breaks down stones and relieves constipation. Raspberries support the female organs and break down mucous. Olive oil is a good laxative and breaks down liver and gallstones for removal from the body. Raw honey has antiseptic properties and is good for coughs and sore throats when mixed with lemon juice and warm water.

Ingredients:
1/4 cup raw cider vinegar
1/4 cup cold-pressed olive oil
3/4 cup fresh raspberries
4 tablespoons raw honey
1 cup water

Blend all ingredients and serve.
Yield: Approximately 1 pint.

Raw Crackers
(from the kitchen of Linda Ruff)

These crackers make a good travel food. The flaxseeds are an excellent source of omega-3's. The onion stabilizes blood sugars and fights parasites. The celery is full of electrolytes, and sage is good for the skin and scalp and fights colds, fevers, and headaches.

Ingredients:
1 large chopped onion
2 ribs of chopped celery
2 teaspoons dried sage
1 cup water
2 cups ground flaxseed
Himalayan salt, if tolerated

Blend first 4 ingredients together. Add ground flaxseed to blended mix until slimy. Spread thinly on dehydrator sheets. Shape into squares or triangles and sprinkle with Himalayan salt, if tolerated. Dehydrate to desired moistness or crispness. Crackers will need to be turned after approximately 8 hours.

Yield: 30-50 crackers.

VARIATION: For flavor variations try substituting other spices such as garlic, oregano, and basil.

Raw Applesauce
(adapted from the kitchen of the Ann Wigmore
Natural Health Institute)

It is absolutely amazing how good fresh raw applesauce can taste. Apples, especially when green, provide malic acid which is great for breaking down liver stones and gallstones and flushing them out of the body. Apples also provide pectin which is excellent for sweeping the colon of impactions and other matter and prevents protein putrefaction in the gut. Pectin also removes heavy metals and radioactive materials from the body. Cinnamon strengthens and energizes body tissues while stabilizing blood sugar levels.

Ingredients:
4 or 5 apples
1/4-1/2 teaspoon cinnamon

Blend apples and cinnamon with enough water for blending until smooth and creamy. Raw honey to taste may be added for tart green apples.

Yield: 1-2 cups.

Fruit Pizza
(from the kitchen of Linda Ruff)

This pretty dish decorated with raw fruit is tempting to all, including omnivores. Its beneficial properties are highest when the raw fruits are fresh from farmer's markets and local growers. This dish provides plenty of fiber, omega-3's, carotenoids and other antioxidants, and loads of beneficial phytochemicals that promote good health for everyone, including diabetics.

Ingredients:
1 1/2 teaspoons cinnamon
1 1/2 cups English walnuts
1 date, soaked overnight in
  water to cover
OR 1 tablespoon raw honey
Plain Cheesy White Sauce
Variety of sliced colored fruits,
  (kiwi, papaya, peaches,
  blueberries, strawberries,
  banana, etc.)

In a food processor or Vita-Mix blend the cinnamon and English walnuts until crumbly. Then add the dates and soak water to form a stiff dough. Water may need to be added. Shape the dough on a pizza pan. Spread Cheesy White Sauce over the crust and decorate with fruits.
Yield: 1 9-10" pie.

VARIATION: Try pressing the walnut crust into a pie plate. Add a fruit such as strawberries, cherries, blackberries, or other to the Cheesy White Sauce and pour into the crust to make a creamy fruit pie. Decorate with any remaining fruit.

Blueberry Cobbler
(from the kitchen of Linda Ruff)

The high antioxidant content of blueberries strengthen the eyes and support good night vision, fight infection, and are a good laxative. The ground flaxseeds thicken the blueberry juice and create the filler. Flaxseeds are a complete protein and high in lignans which fight breast cancer. Along with flaxseeds, the English walnuts are a good source of omega-3 fatty acids and lubricate the digestive tract for easy elimination. The fiber and natural sugars in dates make a far better sweetener and provide long-lasting energy without the letdown of refined sugars. The lemon juice picks up the flavor and acts as a preservative, and cinnamon helps to relieve intestinal gas.

Ingredients:
4-5 cups fresh or fresh-frozen wild blueberries
1/4 cup ground flaxseeds
1-2 tablespoons fresh squeezed lemon juice
2 teaspoons cinnamon
1 1/2 cups English walnuts
3/4 cup dates

Combine and stir by hand the blueberries, lemon juice, cinnamon, and ground flaxseeds until well mixed and pour into a casserole bowl or dish. Grind the English walnuts in a Vita-Mix or food processor until fine. Then grind the dates into the nuts until thoroughly mixed. Sprinkle the walnut-date mixture over the top of the blueberry mixture to make a crumbly topping.
Yield: 4-5 servings.

NOTE: Other fruits such as blackberries, apples, or cherries may be substituted for blueberries.

Strawberry Crumble Pudding
(from the kitchen of Linda Ruff)

This pudding is so simple to make and tastes so good. Strawberries have cancer fighting properties and promote peristalsis. Both the flaxseeds and walnuts pack the essential omega-3 fatty acid. The dates sweeten without an energy letdown.

Ingredients:
1 cup fresh strawberries
1/4-1/2 cup ground flaxseeds
1 cup English walnuts
2 dates

Blend the strawberries and pour into 2 or 3 pudding dishes. Stir in the ground flaxseeds until well mixed. In a food processor or Vita-Mix grind the walnuts until crumbly. Add the dates and blend until mixture is crumbly. Sprinkle on top of puddings and refrigerate until mixture thickens.
Yield: 2-3 servings.

VARIATION: For a delicious banana pudding, eliminate the ground flaxseeds and substitute frozen bananas for the strawberries. Add sliced bananas in the blended pudding and sprinkle with the walnut date crumbs.

Apple and Date Cookies
(from the kitchen of Linda Sanders-Sheer)

These cookies provide a delicious alternative at snack time and are loaded with fiber. The potassium in the bananas nourishes the brain and nervous system. The apples provide pectin which clears out the digestive tract and eliminates toxins. Coconut carries iodine, and English walnuts provide omega-3 fatty acids, adding a rich flavor. Vanilla can be soothing to the stomach and adds flavor, and dates are a natural sweetener with fiber that sustain an individual throughout daily tasks without a letdown.

Ingredients:
2 1/2-3 cups dates, soaked overnight
  in filtered water
4 or 5 apples, chopped
4 or 5 bananas, sliced
3 cups unsweetened coconut
2 cups or more of English walnuts
2 teaspoons to 1 tablespoon vanilla

Combine ingredients and stir well. Dehydrate for 1 1/2 to 2 days depending upon desired dryness and climate.
Yield: Approximately 4 dozen cookies.

NOTE: Serve the mixture without dehydration in a bowl for a delicious dessert. Note the difference in the flavors of the dessert and the dehydrated cookies.

Egyptian Candy
(from *Purely Delicious* magazine, fall 2007)

According to this informative magazine, this delicious recipe was found on a fragment of an old Egyptian clay pot. This healthy candy provides omega-3's from the walnuts and healthy sweeteners from the dates and raw honey. Both cinnamon and cardamom warm the body, and cardamom helps sharpen the mind. Raw honey has vitamins and minerals not found in refined sugars, and unpasteurized almonds support nerve and bone strength.

Ingredients:
1 cup ground English walnuts
1 cup fresh dates
1/2 teaspoon ground cinnamon
1/2 teaspoon ground cardamom
Small amount of warm raw honey
1/2 cup ground unpasteurized almonds

Grind the English walnuts in a food processor or Vita-Mix until fine. Make a paste of dates in a Vita-Mix or food processor. Combine walnuts and dates and stir in spices. Roll into balls and gently coat with warmed honey. Roll in ground almonds. Keep refrigerated or frozen until ready to serve.
Yield: About 1 dozen.

NOTE: Almonds are high in arginine which may promote cold sores and herpes viruses. For anyone prone to these infections, lysine prevents cold sores and infections. Good sources of lysine, which is destroyed with cooking, are legumes, fruits, and vegetables.

NOTE: The federal government now requires almonds to be pasteurized. The two processes of pasteurization are 1) steam heat the life from the almonds or 2) inject a chemical into the almonds. To obtain unpasteurized almonds, purchase them directly from an almond grower.

Cinnamon Pears
(from the kitchen of Linda Ruff)

Dehydrated cinnamon pears are a sweet delicacy that taste just like cinnamon rolls. Actually pears are a better cleanser of the body than apples. They provide more pectin which breaks down and cleanses the digestive tract, liver, and gallbladder.

Ingredients:
4 or 5 pears
Cinnamon to taste

Thinly slice the pears and sprinkle with cinnamon on both sides. Dehydrate for several days, depending on thickness of slices.
Yield: 1-2 cups.

NOTE: The best pears for this recipe are those harvested in the fall fresh from under a tree and allowed to ripen to a pretty golden yellow color full of fresh juice.

Resources

The following can be contacted for more information on raw foods and the Living Foods Lifestyle®.

Ann Wigmore Foundation®
P. O. Box 398
San Fidel, New Mexico 87049
505-552-0595
www.annwigmore.com
www.wigmore.org
www.livingfoodsgardenvillage.com
drannwigmore@gmail.com

This is the first reTREAT founded by Ann Wigmore in 1963 in Boston, Massachusetts. Originally called the Hippocrates Health Institute, the name later changed to the Ann Wigmore Foundation, Inc. and then relocated to New Mexico after Wigmore's death. The Foundation offers a ten day retreat of cleansing and healing and shares the teachings of the Living Foods Lifestyle® with original classes that Wigmore taught.

Ann Wigmore Natural Health Institute, Inc.
P.O. Box 429
Rincon, Puerto Rico 00677-0429
Tel.:   787-868-6307
FAX: 787-868-2430
www.annwigmore.org
info@annwigmore.org
This is the second retreat established by Ann Wigmore in 1990, where I had the privilege of working and furthering my studies in health and healing. Both centers have wonderful, sincere, and LIVE-icated teachers and staff.

Both the Ann Wigmore Natural Health Institute, Inc. and the Ann Wigmore Foundation® are the only two centers authorized to use the trademarks.

Victoria Boutenko
Raw Family
Ashland, Oregon
www.rawfamily.com
Victoria, her husband Igor, their son Sergei, and daughter Valya came
from Russia only to acquire in three years the debilitating diseases that
are prevalent in America. They turned their health around by adopting
a totally raw vegan diet. Since then, they have authored several books
which tell of their inspiring journey, including *Raw Family, 12 Steps to
Raw Foods, Eating Without Heating,* and *Green for Life.* These
entertaining books are full of wit and humor along with excellent raw
vegan recipes.

Lillian Holliger
Martha Paulin
Certified Colon Hydrotherapists
Lillian B. Holliger Inc.
4010 Dupont Circle, Suite 518
Louisville, Kentucky 40207-4888
502-893-2006
www.lillianholliger.com
t.holliger@insightbb.com
I take all of my clients to the chuckly, happy office of Lillian and
Martha because the clients are always extremely happy after their
sessions. Based upon the needs of the client Lillian and Martha
incorporate reflexology, acupressure, Reiki, and other modalities
to relax and facilitate ease of release during the session.

The Grass Shack
Kim Hajduk
Westfield, Indiana
317-714-1734
www.TheGrassShack.com
Kim grows and delivers or ships organic wheatgrass, buckwheat
sprouts, sunflower sprouts, and other microgreens to clients and major
supermarkets on request.

Renee Janette Bogard, E-RYT 200
Certified Experienced Yoga Teacher
Certified Usui Reiki Master/Teacher
Certified Raw Vegan and Living Foods Facilitator
Sedona, Arizona and surrounding area
520-401-1662
www.EssentialElements.ws
Renee instructs raw foods classes and therapeutic yoga in both group
and private classes. She also leads yoga retreats, sells prepared raw
gourmet foods, and offers Reiki treatments and attunements.

Linda Sheer, B.S., R.N., CMTA
Founder of Center of Awakened Health (COAH)
264 East Indiana Avenue
Southern Pines, North Carolina 28387
910-695-1515
www.awakenedhealth.net
The Center of Awakened Health offers 2-day, 5-day, and 12-day
programs as well as hourly appointments designed to help those with
life threatening illnesses or simply for those wishing to learn more
about good health. Linda, who studied under the tutelage of Dr. Ann
Wigmore, and her staff use healing raw foods as well as metabolic
typing, Quantum Reflex Analysis, and many other modalities to
promote health and healing.

References

Chapter 1 – Mother Nature Knows Best

1. Ann Wigmore. *Our Precious Pets.* New York: Copen Press, 1987, pp. 67-69.

2. Ann Wigmore. *Why Suffer?* Wayne, New Jersey: Avery Publishing Group, Inc., 1985, pp. 78-84.

Chapter 3 – What Are Raw and Living Foods?

1. A. L. Rauma et al. "Antioxidant Status in Long-Term Adherents to a Strict Uncooked Vegan Diet." *The American Journal of Clinical Nutrition,* 62:6, December 1995, 1221-1227.

2. O. Hanninen et al. "Antioxidants in Vegan Diet and Rheumatic Disorders." *Toxicology,* 155:1-3, November 30, 2000, 45-53.

3. M. T. Nenonen et al. "Uncooked, Lactobacilli-Rich, Vegan Food and Rheumatoid Arthritis." *British Journal of Rheumatology,* 37:3, March 1998, 274-281.

4. M. S. Donaldson et al. "Fibromyalgia Syndrome Improved Using a Mostly Raw Vegetarian Diet: An Observational Study." *BMC Complimentary and Alternative Medicine,* 1:7, Epub September 26, 2001

5. www.kirlian.com/currentkirlian.htm

6. B. Jensen, *Foods That Heal,* New York: Avery Publishing Group, 1993, 77.

7. Dr. Edward Howell. *Enzyme Nutrition: The Food Enzyme Concept.* Wayne, New Jersey: Avery Publishing Group, Inc., 1985, pp. 2-7 .

8. Ibid, 81.

Chapter 4 – Ode to Green Foods

1. Ed Davis, N.D., Bremen, Kentucky, personal interview, January 29, 2012.

2. B. Jensen, *Foods That Heal,* New York: Avery Publishing Group, 1993, 26.

3. K. M. Van De Graaff and S. I. Fox. *Concepts of Human Anatomy and Physiology, 4ᵗʰ ed.* William C. Brown Publishers, 1995, 551.

4. Ed Davis, N.D., Bremen, Kentucky, personal interview, January 29, 2012.

5. Raw Family Newsletter, "Green Smoothies for Diabetics," 9/10/10.

6. A. Schluter et al. "The Chlorophyll-Derived Metabolite Phytanic Acid Induces White Adipocyte Differentiation." *International Journal of Obesity and Related Metabolic Disorders: Journal of the International Association for the Study of Obesity.* 26:9, September 2002, 1277-80.

7. J. Y. Dong et al. "Magnesium Intake and Risk of Type 2 Diabetes: Meta-Analysis of Prospective Cohort Studies." *Diabetes Care,* 34:9, September 2011, 2116-2122.

8. Mde. L. Lima et al. "The Effect of Magnesium Supplementation in Increasing Doses on the Control of Type 2 Diabetes." *Diabetes Care,* 21:5, May 1998, 682-686.

9. D. King et al. "Dietary Magnesium and C-reactive Protein Levels." *Journal of the American College of Nutrition,* 24(3), 2005, 166-171.

10. 2011 National Diabetes Fact Sheet. Center for Disease Control. Accessible at: cdc.gov/media/releases/2011/p0126_diabetes.html.

11. A. R. Battersby. "Biosynthesis of the Pigments of Life." *Journal of Natural Products.* 51:4, July-August 1988, 629-642.

12. Ibid.

13. M. C. Nahata et al. "Effect of Chlorophyllin on Urinary Odor in Incontinent Geriatric Patients." *Drug Intelligence and Clinical Pharmacy,* 17:10, 1983, 732-734.

14. C. Y. Hsu et al. "Effects of Chlorophyll-Related Compounds on Hydrogen Peroxide Induced DNA Damage within Human Lymphocytes." *Journal of Agricultural and Food Chemistry,* 53:7, April 2005, 2746-2750.

15. A. Yoshida et al. "Therapeutic Effect of Chlorophyll-a in the Treatment of Patients with Chronic Pancreatitis." *Gastroenterologia Japonica,* 15:1, 1980, 49-61.

16. A. Jankowski et al. "Synergistic Action of Photosensitizers and Normal Human Serum in a Bactericidal Process. I. Effect of Chlorophylls." *Acta Microbiologica Polonica,* 52:4, 2003, 373-378.

17. S. S. Kumar et al. "Effect of Chlorophyllin Against Oxidative Stress in Splenic Lymphocytes in Vitro and in Vivo." *Biochimica et Biophysuca Acta,* 1672:2, May 3, 2004, 100-111.

18. S. Chernomorsky et al. "Effect of Dietary Chlorophyll Derivatives on Mutagenesis and Tumor Cell Growth." *Teratogenesis, Carcinogenesis, and Mutagenesis, "* 19:5, 1999, 313-322.

19. M. A. Moors et al. "A Role for Complement Receptor-Like Molecules in Iron Acquisition by Candida Albicans." *The Journal of Experimental Medicine,* 175:6, June 1, 1992, 1643-1651.

20. E. Kaliviotis and M. Yianneskis. "Fast Response Characteristics of Red Blood Cell Aggregation." *Biorheology,* 45:6, 2008, 639-649.

21. C. Wei et al. "Effects of Psychological Stress on Serum Iron and Erythropoiesis." *International Journal of Hematology,* 88:1, July 2008, 52-56.

22. A. Sanchez et al. "Role of Sugars in Human Neutrophilic Phagocytosis." *American Journal of Clinical Nutrition,* 26:11, November 1973, 1180-1184.

23. L. Nizzetto et al. "Seasonality of the Air-Forest Canopy Exchange of Persistent Organic Pollutants." *Environmental Science and Technology,* 42: 23, December 1, 2008, 8778-8783.

Chapter 5 – Raw Juices for Healing

1. Y. L. Lee et al. "Antibacterial Activity of Vegetables and Juices." *Nutrition,* 19:11-12, November-December 2003, 994-996.

2. M. C. de Castillo et al. "Bactericidal Activity of Lemon Juice and Lemon Derivatives against Vibrio cholera." *Biological and Pharmaceutical Bulletin.,* 23:10, October 2000, 1235-1238.

3. C. H. Ruxton et al. "Can Pure Fruit and Vegetable Juices Protect Against Cancer and Cardiovascular Disease Too? A Review of the Evidence." *International Journal of Food Sciences and Nutrition,* 57:3-4, May-June 2006, 249-272.

4. A. S. Potter et al. "Drinking Carrot Juice Increases Total Antioxidant Status and Decreases Lipid Peroxidation in Adults." *Nutrition Journal,* September 24, 2011, 10, 96.

5. R. Edenharder et al. "Protection by Beverages, Fruits, Vegetables, Herbs, and Flavonoids against Genotoxicity of 2-acetylaminofluorene and 2-amino-1-methyl-6-phenylimidazo[4,5-b] pyridine (PhIP) in Metabolically Competent V79 Cells." *Mutation Research,* 521:1-2, November 26, 2002, 57-72.

6. V. Krajka-Kuzniak et al. "Modulation of Rat Hepatic and Kidney Phase II Enzymes by Cabbage Juices: Comparison with the Effects of Indole-3-Carbinol and Phenethyl Isothiocyanate." *British Journal of Nutrition,* 105:6, March 2011, 816-826.

7. A. S. Potter et al. "Drinking Carrot Juice Increases Total Antioxidant Status and Decreases Lipid Peroxidation in Adults." *Nutrition Journal,* September 24 2011, 10, 96.

8. R. G. Cutler. "Carotenoids and Retinol: Their Possible Importance in Determining Longevity of Primate Species." *Proceedings of the National Academy of Sciences of the United States of America,* 81:23, December 1984, 7627-7631.

9. D. R. Davis et al. "Changes in USDA Food Composition Data for 43 Garden Crops, 1950 to 1999." *Journal of the American College of Nutrition,* 23:6, December 2004, 669-682.

10. M. S. Fan et al. "Evidence of Decreasing Mineral Density in Wheat Grain over the Last 160 Years." *Journal of Trace Elements in Medicine and Biology,* 22:4, 2008, 315-324.

Chapter 6 – The Many Uses of Wheatgrass Juice

1. Ann Wigmore. *Why Suffer?* Wayne, New Jersey: Avery Publishing Group, 1985, 129-130.

2. R. K. Marawaha et al. "Wheat Grass Juice Reduces Transfusion Requirement in Patients with Thalassemia Major: A Pilot Study." *Indian Pediatrics,* 41:7, July 2004, 716-720.

3. D. R. Choudhary et al. "Effect of Wheat Grass Therapy on Transfusion Requirement in Beta- Thalassemia Major." *Indian Journal of Pediatrics,* 76:4, April 2009, 375-376.

4. S. Kothari et al. "Hypolipidemic Effect of Fresh Triticum Aestivum (Wheat) Grass Juice in Hypercholesterolemic Rats." *Acta Poloniae Pharmaceutica,* 68:2, March 2011, 291-294.

5. E. Ben-Arye, "Wheat Grass Juice in the Treatment of Active Distal Ulcerative Colitis: A Randomized Double-Blind Placebo-Controlled Trial." *Scandinavian Journal of Gastroenterology,* 37:4, April 2002, 444-449.

6. N. B. Alitheen et al. "Cytotoxic Effects of Commercial Wheatgrass and Fiber towards Human Acute Promyelocytic Leukemia Cells (HL60)." *Pakistan Journal of Pharmaceutical Sciences,* 24:3, July 2011, 243-250.

7. G. Bar-Sela et al. "Wheat Grass Juice May Improve Hematological Toxicity Related to Chemotherapy in Breast Cancer Patients: A Pilot Study." *Nutrition and Cancer,* 58:1, 2007, 43-48.

Chapter 7 – Sprouts and Nutrition

1. Ann Wigmore. *Our Precious Pets,* New York: Copen Press, 1987, 13.

2. C. Rodriguez et al. "Total Chemically Available (Free and Intrachain) Lysine and Furosine in Pea, Bean, and Lentil Sprouts." *Journal of Agricultural and Food Chemistry,* 55:25, December 2007, 10275-10280.

3. "Protein Content." *Living Foods Lifestyle^{TM}: Ann Wigmore Natural Health Institute.* Puerto Rico, 148.

4. Ann Wigmore. *The Hippocrates Diet and Health Program.* Wayne, New Jersey: Avery Publishing Group, Inc., 1984, 72-75.

5. M. Moriyama and K. Oba. "Sprouts as Antioxidant Food Resources and Young People's Taste For Them." *Biofactors,* 21:1-4, 2004, 247-249.

6. M. Murashima et al. "Phase 1 Study of Multiple Biomarkers for Metabolism and Oxidative Stress after One-Week Intake of Broccoli Sprouts." *Biofactors,* 22:1-4, 2004, 271-275.

7. M. Akhlaghi and B. Bandy. "Dietary Broccoli Sprouts Protect Against Myocardial Oxidative Damage and Cell Death during Ischemia-Reperfusion." *Plant Foods for Human Nutrition,* 65:3, September 2010, 193-199.

8. R. Munday et al. "Inhibition of Urinary Bladder Carcinogenesis by Broccoli Sprouts." *Cancer Research,* 68:5, March 1, 2008, 1593-1600.

9. J. W. Fahey et al. "Broccoli Sprouts: an Exceptionally Rich Source of Inducers of Enzymes That Protect Against Chemical Carcinogens." *Proceedings of the National Academy of Sciences of the United States of America*, 94:19, September 16, 1997, 10367-10372.

10. S. Ishii et al. "Anti-Inflammatory Effect of Buckwheat Sprouts in Lipopolysaccharide-Activated Human Colon Cancer Cells and Mice." *Bioscience, Biotechnology, and Biochemistry,* 72:12, December 2008, 3148-3157.

11. A. Yanaka et al. "Dietary Sulforaphane-Rich Broccoli Sprouts Reduce Colonization and Attenuate Gastritis in Helicobacter Pylori-Infected Mice and Humans." *Cancer Prevention Research,* 2:4, April 2009, 353-360.

12. R. Randhir et al. "Phenolics, Their Antioxidant and Antimicrobial Activity in Dark Germinated Fenugreek Sprouts in Response to Peptide and Phytochemical Elicitors." *Asia Pacific Journal Of Clinical Nutrition,* 13:3, 2004, 295-307.

13. Dr. Edward Howell. *Enzyme Nutrition: The Food Enzyme Concept.* Wayne, New Jersey: Avery Publishing Group, Inc., 1985, 120.

Chapter 8 – Detoxification – The Right Hand of Living Foods

1. Physicians Committee for Responsible Medicine. "Truth in Advertising: PCRM Fights for Biohazard Labeling on Meat." *Good Medicine,* Winter 2002, 6-7.

2. Environmental Working Group, http://www.ewg.org/sites/bodyburden1/findings.php.

3. Environmental Working Group, http://www.ewg.org/dioxin/research.

4. H. Farah and J. Buzby. "U.S. Food Consumption Up 16 Percent Since 1970." *Amber Waves,* Nov. 2005, www.ers.usda.gov/AmberWaves/November05/Findings/usfoodconsumption.htm

5. D. R. Davis et al. "Changes in USDA Food Composition Data for 43 Garden Crops, 1950 to 1999." *Journal of the American College of Nutrition,* 23:6, December 2004, 669-682.

6. B. Jensen. *Dr. Jensen's Guide to Better Bowel Care,* New York: Avery, 1999, 36.

7. N. Walker, D.Sc., Ph.D. *Colon Health: the Key to a Vibrant Life,* Phoenix: O'Sullivan Woodside and Company, 1979, 6-14.

8. R. Gray, *The Colon Health Handbook,* 12th ed., Reno: Emerald Publishing, Dec. 1991, 7-14.

9. Ibid, 12-13.

10. N. Walker, D.Sc., Ph.D. *Colon Health: the Key to a Vibrant Life,* Phoenix: O'Sullivan Woodside and Company, 1979, 7.

11. Ibid, 13.

12. R. Gray, *The Colon Health Handbook,* 12th ed., Reno: Emerald Publishing, Dec. 1991, 23.

13. P. Christensen et al. "Long-Term Outcome and Safety of Transanal Irrigation for Constipation and Fetal Incontinence." *Diseases of the Colon and Rectum,* 52:2, February 2009, 286-292.

14. N. J. Taffinder et al. "Retrograde Commercial Colonic Hydrotherapy." *Colorectal Disease: The Official Journal of the Association of Coloproctology of Great Britain and Ireland,* 6:4, July 2004, 258-260.

15. R. Gray, *The Colon Health Handbook,* 12th ed., Reno: Emerald Publishing, Dec. 1991, 14.

16. Ibid.

Chapter 9 – Deeper Cleansing

1. B. Jensen, *Foods That Heal,* New York: Avery Publishing Group, 1993, 26.

2. N. Walker, D.Sc., Ph.D. *Diet and Salad,* Phoenix: O'Sullivan Woodside and Company, 1971, 140.

3. B. Jensen, *Foods That Heal,* New York: Avery Publishing Group, 1993, 79-80, 170-171.

4. Ibid.

5. R. Gray, *The Colon Health Handbook,* 12th ed., Reno: Emerald Publishing, Dec. 1991, 13.

6. N. Walker, D.Sc., Ph.D. *Colon Health: the Key to a Vibrant Life,* Phoenix: O'Sullivan Woodside and Company, 1979, 22.

7. S. U. Jeong and S. K. Lee. "Obesity and Gallbladder Diseases." *The Korean Journal of Gastroenterology,* 59:1, 2012, 27-34.

8. N. Walker, D.Sc., Ph.D. *Colon Health: the Key to a Vibrant Life,* Phoenix: O'Sullivan Woodside and Company, 1979, 125-127.

9. R. Gray, *The Colon Health Handbook,* 12th ed., Reno: Emerald Publishing, Dec. 1991, 24.

10. C. Ottley. "Food and Mood." *Nursing Standard (Royal College of Nursing - Great Britain),* 15:2, September 27-October 3, 2000, 46-52.

11. A. Sanchez-Villegas et al. "Fast-Food and Commercial Baked Goods Consumption and the Risk of Depression." *Public Health Nutrition,* 15:3, March 2012, 424-432.

12. M. E. Vollrath et al. "Children and Eating. Personality and Gender Are Associated with Obesogenic Food Consumption and Overweight in 6- to 12-year-olds." *Appetite*, 58:3, March 15, 2012, 1113-1117.

Chapter 10 – Emotional Cleansing

1. K. M. Van De Graaff and S. I. Fox. *Concepts of Human Anatomy and Physiology, 4th ed.* William C. Brown Publishers, 1995, 626.
2. Ibid, 625.

3. B. Jensen, *Foods That Heal,* New York: Avery Publishing Group, 1993, 21.

4. Ibid, 56-57.

5. A. Sanchez et al. "Role of Sugars in Human Neutrophilic Phagocytosis." *American Journal of Clinical Nutrition,* 26:11, November 1973, 1180-1184.

6. B. Jensen, *Foods That Heal,* New York: Avery Publishing Group, 1993, 21.

Chapter 11 – A Joyful Way of Life

1. B. Jensen, *Foods That Heal,* New York: Avery Publishing Group, 1993, 68-69.

2. Leola Brooks, Co-Director of the Ann Wigmore Natural Health Institute, Rincon, Puerto Rico, Interview, 11/15/10.

About the Author

Linda Ruff is a registered dietitian who worked at the Ann Wigmore Natural Health Institute in Puerto Rico. There she taught classes and furthered her studies in health and nutrition by learning of cleansing and healing through raw and living foods.

Linda combines her clinical experience as a dietitian with an understanding of the body's processes and how the body is affected by various properties, types, and preparations of foods. She provides personalized programs and on-going coaching using raw and living foods to eliminate disease as well as maintain good health. Her program is very successful for clients with energy deficits, obesity, irritable bowel and other colon issues, candida and fungal infections, arthritis, cancer, and many other health issues. She currently consults, teaches, and lectures throughout the Midwest.

Linda can be reached at the following:
P.O. Box 6624
Evansville, Indiana 47719
livingfoodsdietitian@gmail.com
www.livingfoodsdietitian.com

To order books, contact her at her e-mail address
or contact the publisher at: birdbrainproductions@ymail.com

Linda Lamar Ruff, R.D.

The authentic work of Linda Ruff adds a breath of freshness into the subject of raw foods. The author starts her book with impressive testimonials from people who restored their health by practicing a raw foods diet, gathered during her work at the Ann Wigmore Natural Health Institute in Puerto Rico. Ruff shares inspiring stories about Ann Wigmore's life and how her teaching continues to heal people. The sincerity and passion of the book add strength to the message. Many true life anecdotes and observations make it an engaging read.   - *Victoria Boutenko,*
Author of numerous raw foods publications

Linda Ruff was a dedicated student of the Living Foods Lifestyle® as taught by the Ann Wigmore Natural Health Institute in Puerto Rico. While a student, she adopted the lifestyle without reservation and practiced it with patience and love. As a student and later as a returning graduate, Linda showed great interest in helping people. While at the Institute, she used her own healing experiences to inspire and motivate others. She also listened to them and collected their information.

Today Linda is still interested in helping people. By using the information previously collected at the Institute, she developed her own detox program. Many people may find Linda's approach using raw foods to be very effective as a transition tool from cooked to living foods as well as a useful step towards healing.   - *Lalita Salas, Co-Director,*
The Ann Wigmore Natural Health Institute
Author, Candida Health Through Living Foods

Blessings and Healing to our whole nation and Universe is achieved through the great service of such wonderful leaders as Linda Ruff, who graciously seeks to be in the service to the Oneness of All Life. Anyone who puts forth a book such as this is clearly a Way Shower!

All the more POWER to the blessings that we all may receive as we one by one and two by two move on in healing our bodies with the One Blueprint that Dr. Ann Wigmore, our Mother of Wheatgrass and Living Foods, produced. Hurrah! and Praises!!! Let us All live in true Live-ication - not dedication.   - *Susan L. Lavendar, Director,*
The Ann Wigmore Foundation

Other works published by Vita Aeterna Advanced Wellness Books

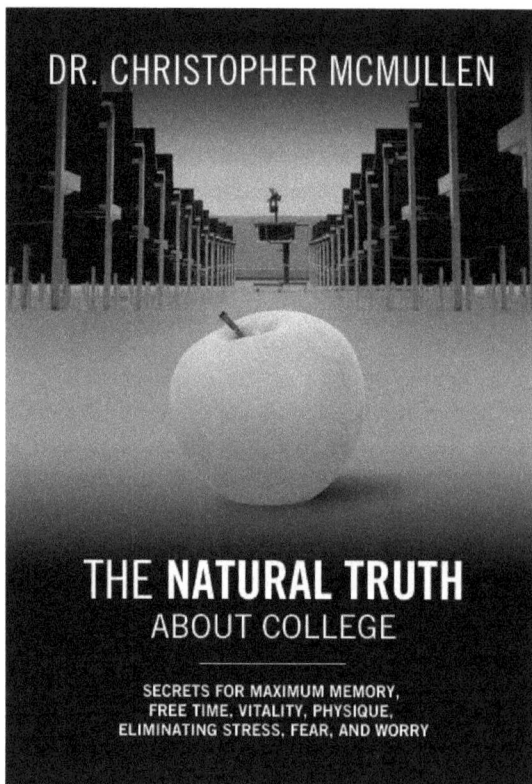

"Every college student needs to read and heed
the great HEALTH advice in The Natural Truth about College!
It will help you for the rest of your life!"
- C. Norman Shealy, M.D., Ph.D., Founder of the American Holistic
Medical Association, President, Holos Institutes of Health

The Natural Truth about College:
Secrets for Maximum Memory, Free Time, Vitality, Physique,
Eliminating Stress, Fear, and Worry
By
Dr. Chris McMullen

Available on Kindle and Amazon.com

www.ingramcontent.com/pod-product-compliance
Lightning Source LLC
Chambersburg PA
CBHW031857090426
42741CB00005B/531